GOT DISCIPLINE?

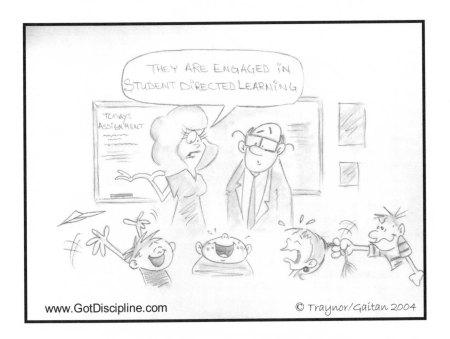

RESEARCH-BASED PRACTICES FOR MANAGING STUDENT BEHAVIOR

Patrick Traynor, Ph.D.

University of California, Riverside

Elizabeth Traynor, M.D.

Neurologist, Consulting Author

ii

Library of Congress Cataloging-in-Publication Data
Traynor, P. L., 1963-
    Got discipline? Researched-Based Practices for Managing Student Behavior / P. L. Traynor
            p.   cm.
    Includes bibliographical references and index
    ISBN 0-9765618-0-9 (pbk.)
    1. Classroom management—United States 2. Discipline—United States 3. School discipline—United States 4. Classroom Discipline—United States
I. Title

Additional copies of this book are available at www.GotDiscipline.com, Atlas Books, Barnes & Noble, or at a favorite online or local bookstore.

A Product of
EduThinkTank Research Group
Irvine, CA
www.EduThinkTank.com

Printed in the U.S.A. by
BookMasters
2541 Ashland Rd.
Mansfield, OH 44805
Ph.: 800-537-6727

TABLE OF CONTENTS

ACKNOWLEDGEMENTS

The author wishes to acknowledge and thank the following persons for their direct, indirect, professional, or personal contributions to this work.

Flora Ida Ortiz, Ph.D., Professor, UCR
John McNeil, Ph.D., Professor Emeritus, UCLA
Douglas Mitchell, Ph.D., Professor, UCR
Gerald Gaitan, Cartoonist
Mary Beth Richardson, Nationally Board Certified Teacher
Kathleen Penrice, Teacher
James French, Teacher
Alex Thurman, Teacher
Michael Ochs, Teacher
Frank Acosta, Teacher
Bruce Webb, Teacher
And all the participants who have contributed to the case studies herein and a better understanding of classroom management. And finally, the author wishes to acknowledge spouse and consulting author, Elizabeth N. Traynor, M.D. and their two sons, Patrick and Christopher.

PREFACE

This book describes current research-based practices for managing student behavior in today's school environment. Actual episodes from case studies precede each practice, are presented in a comprehensible framework, and illustrate the virtues of effective practices and the pitfalls of others. The author, Dr. Traynor, also discusses interacting with parents, Attention Deficit Hyperactivity Disorder (ADHD), antisocial behavior, the first day of school, the office referral, and customer service. *Got Discipline? Research-Based Practices for Managing Student Behavior* is suitable for all people responsible for school age children including teachers, student teachers, substitute teachers, supervisors of teachers, babysitters, coaches, parents, and other child leaders.

PART I   THE CLASSROOM MANAGEMENT SPECTRUM

Mr. Alfred casually stood by the door greeting students prior to class. Some entered laughing, conversing jokingly and a couple playfully shouted across the room. One student exclaimed in a comical voice, "Whatchya gunna to do now?" Another asked urgently, "Mr. Alfred, Mr. Alfred, can I go to the bathroom really, really quickly?" One boy strongly kicked a backpack that was on the floor in a teasing but agitated manner. Mr. Alfred did not react to any of the ruckus inside the classroom. The beginning bell rang and Mr. Alfred announced the beginning of class, "Okay ladies and gentlemen . . ." A student interrupted with a question to which Mr. Alfred responded, "Don't worry about that. We're not going to do that. I'll tell you what we're going to do." Another boy began to carry a student project to his seat. Mr. Alfred addressed him, "Chris Alexander, that's not yours. Okay?" Despite Mr. Alfred's announcement of the beginning of class, several students continued conversing and several were wondering around the room. Mr. Alfred responded to the noise, "Shhh." One student remarked, "It's stupid." Mr. Alfred announced, "Ladies and gentlemen, in your seats, I'm taking roll!" However, the ruckus continued.

   Children do not naturally order themselves in groups of 20 to 40 under the guidance of an unfamiliar adult in close quarters, behave orderly, and engage in learning. Behavior in today's classroom needs to be effectively managed for productive learning to occur. Cusick (1992) attests, "Control is the major issue and always at the center of the student-teacher relations. Orderly behavior can never be expected; it is always problematic and always requires attention" (p. 46). Brint (1998) affirms, "Classroom order is a precondition for teaching and learning" (p. 260). The inspirational mathematics teacher, Jaime Escalante verifies, "No matter how much money and programs, it won't work – unless they understand respect and discipline in the classroom" (Walker, Colvin, and Ramsey, 1995; p. 437). Research unequivocally confirms classroom order is associated with teacher confidence and higher levels of learning (Coleman, Hoffer, and Kilgore 1982; Newman, Rutter, and Smith, 1989; Traynor, 2002).

CHAPTER

1

Three Approaches
To Classroom Management

Various authors on the subject of classroom management refer to three general approaches toward maintaining classroom order (Dreikers, Grunwald, and Pepper, 1982; Canter and Canter, 1992; Steinberg, Dornbush, and Brown, 1992; Coloroso, 1994; Albert, 1996; Jones, 2000). Although they use a variety of names to label them, the approaches described are essentially the same and are referred to here as lenient, rigid, and moderate (see Traynor, 2004 for a more detailed comparison). A teacher who takes a more laissez-faire approach, has low expectations for student behavior, and allows disruptions to occur characterizes the lenient approach. A teacher who demonstrates little tolerance for student misbehavior, applies coercive practices such as shouting, threats, or unreasonable punishments, and has little or no regard for the students' emotional or educational well-being characterizes the rigid approach. A teacher who demonstrates self-control, consistency, and holds students accountable to a fair set of classroom rules characterizes the moderate approach.

CHAPTER

2

Five Categories of Practices

Traynor (2004) showed how the styles of teachers who were strongly identified with a single approach were related to the three approaches: Lenient, Rigid, and Moderate (Figure 1). Practices belonging to each approach were found to exist on a common continuum that includes five categories of practices. (Figure 1 will be referred to frequently throughout this book. Bookmark this page for easy reference.)

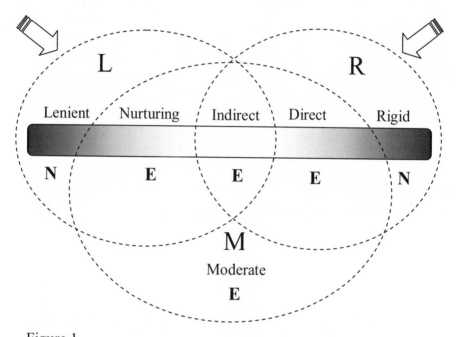

Figure 1
The Classroom Management Spectrum. L = Lenient teachers. R = Rigid teachers. M = Moderate teachers. E = Effective N = Not effective. Arrows = Movement toward more effectiveness. Note: Adapted from Traynor (2004)

The circles in Figure 1 show, for all three approaches, shared and unique practices of teachers strongly identified with a single approach. The dashed quality represents the permeability of the approaches. For example, a teacher strongly identified with the rigid approach, could also demonstrate at least to a limited extent, nurturing practices as the perimeter allows for overlap.

The bar within Figure 1 shows the relationship of the approaches on a common continuum. At the extremes are the ineffective lenient and rigid practices. A teacher with a strong lenient or rigid disposition can readily enact the respective proximate and more effective nurturing or direct intervention practices, as these areas of the continuum are contiguous with the extremes. Conversely, a teacher who possesses either of these extreme dispositions would have difficulty enacting the practices at the opposite extreme and would even have difficulty applying the practices adjacent to the opposite extreme as well, as these areas on the continuum are distant from each other. The continuum quality of the bar also reveals that even a teacher possessing one of the extreme dispositions would find the middle, indirect interventions, accessible, as these practices are not too far from the extremes. The continuum quality also shows that a moderate teacher, who possesses a more central moderate disposition, certainly has the indirect interventions readily accessible and can easily apply both the adjacent nurturing practices and direct interventions. The model also shows that a teacher with a moderate disposition is able to refrain from enacting rigid practices – for the rigid disposition is fairly distant from the moderate disposition on the continuum. Similarly, the moderate teacher is able to avoid being overly lenient, as the lenient and moderate dispositions are also fairly distant from each other.

The bar's black and white gradient also shows the increases in effectiveness of the practices from the extremes of the continuum to the center. The black areas at the extremes indicate ineffective practices and the gray and white areas toward the center indicate effective practices. The practices were evaluated as effective or ineffective using Standard Two of the California Standards for the Teaching Profession (see Appendix) according to Traynor (2004).

The model clearly shows that the moderate approach is the most effective of the three, as it contains only effective practices. A teacher using the moderate approach avoids the ineffective lenient and rigid practices at the extremes of the continuum and can readily apply the effective direct, indirect, and nurturing practices.

The arrows in Figure 1 help show how teachers who are strongly identified with the lenient or rigid approach can increase their overall effectiveness. As the circles encompassing the practices of the lenient or rigid teachers move in the direction of the arrows, their ineffective practices are decreased and the more effective practices are increased. Please see Traynor (2004) for a more complete explanation of dispositions and practices of teachers strongly identified with each approach.

CHAPTER

3   **Perception, Skill, and Attitude**

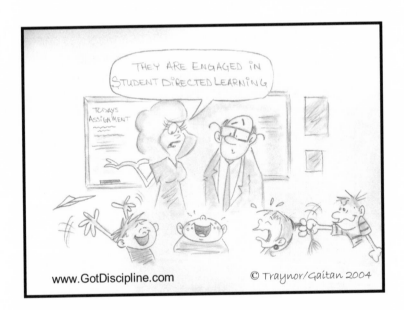

A teacher's ability to implement effective practices depends on (1) ability to perceive maladaptive behavior in the classroom environment, (2) skill in selecting and implementing an appropriate practice, and (3) attitude toward enacting a particular practice. For example, a teacher might have a great attitude toward establishing an effective learning environment but not tend to particular disruptions, as they might not be perceived as detrimental.

Similarly, another teacher might have a good attitude toward maintaining productive order and be able to perceive maladaptive behavior readily in the environment. However, this teacher might not have the skill to select or enact an appropriate classroom order strategy. For example, a well prepared teacher who is aware of the challenges disruptive students pose might not have the assertive skills required to direct students to behave orderly or implement even fair and reasonable consequences.

Also, another teacher might be quite experienced in identifying and enacting appropriate strategies and be able to identify maladaptive behavior readily in the environment. However, knowing that managing classroom behavior is a constant effort that persistently demands attention, this teacher might not wish to devote the time and effort necessary to maintain a highly productive classroom environment. Simply stated, this teacher might not have the proper attitude.

To increase the implementation of effective practices and avoid enactment of ineffective ones, the teacher should examine what is needed: perception, skill, or attitude. If a heightened perception is needed, the descriptions of various scenarios in this book will increase awareness of some of the insidious behaviors naturally present in a group of children. The effectiveness of various responses to those behaviors will also be revealed. If more skill or knowledge is needed, the teacher may of course practice and hone a particular strategy to increase effectiveness. If a better attitude is needed, the descriptions below will put the practices into an organized framework and the teacher will see that the enactment of only a few additional practices will make the difference between an exemplary learning environment and a mediocre one. This teacher will most certainly find a decrease in parent phone calls, "constructive" administrator contacts, and stress.

PART II   Classroom Management Practices

S everal of the most common practices that influence classroom order are illustrated next with descriptions of actual cases. This part of the book is divided into five categories of practices that correspond to the five areas on the continuum model in Figure 1: Lenient, nurturing, indirect, direct, and rigid. Organizing the practices in this manner will provide a useful framework for a classroom teacher, substitute teacher, school site administrator, parent, student teacher, or group leader toward understanding and managing the complex behaviors of groups of school age children.

CATEGORY **1** –

LENIENT PRACTICES

The lenient disposition is at the far left of the Venn
diagram continuum model in Figure 1. Lenient practices
are characterized by geniality and teacher tolerance of
disruptive behavior. Rickman and Hollowell (1981) found these
practices common in their study of student teacher failure. They
found student teachers tend to believe the correct approach to
classroom order is a "laissez-faire" style in which teachers
attempt to become accepted as a peer of their students. Lenient
teachers generally believe acceptance is similar to respect,
which in turn is related to student compliance. However, Grant
(1988) argues that compliance based on friendship and geniality
is not sufficient to motivate students to perform the work
necessary to learn. Cusick (1983) illustrates why the lenient
approach is tempting but not effective:

> "Non-teaching" was one way to deal with a class, not a
> good way according to any learning theory, but a way
> that kept students orderly. No one disobeyed a direction
> that was never given, no one failed to hand in an
> assignment that was never assigned, no one flunked a
> test when there were none, and no student teacher

conflicts, fights or cases of insubordination showed up in the office (p. 55).

From this point forward in Part II, descriptions from actual case studies will introduce and illustrate each practice. Real names, subjects, and other identifying features have been masked for the purpose of keeping participants anonymous.

CHAPTER

4   **Restroom Passes**

M r. Bent was reviewing an assignment with his class and was having his students solve some problems as he walked among them, providing assistance as necessary. A student asked, "Can I go to the bathroom?" Mr. Bent responded, "Can you hold it?" The student answered, "No." Mr. Bent then proposed, "It's up to you." He then proceeded to the front of the class, wrote a message on a piece of paper and gave it to the student. This task consumed approximately 30 seconds of Mr. Bent's time – time otherwise spent on other student interactions.

Disruptions from students needing to use the restroom occur everywhere and create a dilemma for classroom teachers. On one hand, a child having an accident in the classroom clearly must be avoided. The potential loss of dignity is too great to risk. Further, if a teacher unconditionally denies restroom passes to students, the students will perceive the teacher as unfair and parents may complain about the rigid demeanor of the teacher. On the other hand, if a teacher allows any student to use the restroom at will, classroom disruptions from restroom passes will quickly become established as the norm. Additionally, if several teachers in a school allow students to use the restroom whenever they wish, students from different classes will inevitably conspire to get out of class at certain times so that they can be together.

Although no solution to this problem is perfect, effective teachers respond with firm but fair strategies. Some allow any student to use the restroom with the condition that the student spends the amount of time out of class, with the teacher after class. When students realize that they have to sacrifice time after the dismissal bell, they quickly find that passing periods between classes indeed provide sufficient time. Other effective teachers issue one to a few restroom passes each grading period that can be used at any time. Unused restroom passes can be turned in to the teacher at the end of the grading period for extra points. This system provides an incentive, extra points, for students to not use the restroom, yet does not forbid restroom use in the event of a legitimate emergency. If a student depletes the supply of passes, the student must ask the teacher for more, individually. The teacher could then call the parent or work with the individual student, if using the restroom becomes excessive. If the student genuinely has a medical condition or other situation that does not permit restraining for sustained periods of time, extra passes of course would be provided without consequence.

CHAPTER

5

Avoidance

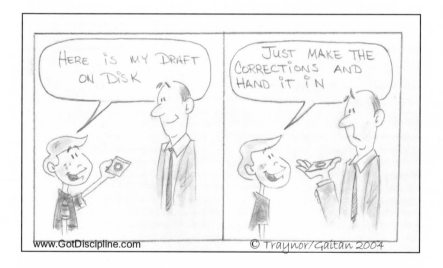

any students were working efficiently, creating a poster of an atom in Mr. Cape's classroom. However, Mr. Cape walked passed one group of students who was talking about basketball, a topic unrelated to their project. They were interjecting humorous comments throughout their conversation. One student responded to another, "Shut up . . . I can shoot. I know who can ball you up!" Another student yelled out to the class, "Heck yeah! Look at this guys!" He then displayed a magazine page of a rock and roll celebrity, Mick Jagger, who had his mouth wide open. Several students laughed at this student's antics and the picture. Mr. Cape did not intervene or prompt any of these students to work more efficiently. A student yelled from the back of the room, "Mr. Cape!" Mr. Cape did not respond. Mr. Cape announced, "Alright guys. We have about ten minutes. We need to clean up in five and if you're not done, you need to finish up at home. I'm up and about correcting papers." A girl threw a crumpled paper from approximately 10 feet from a waste can across Mr. Cape's desk. One student said jokingly, "Hurry it's an emergency. Hurry it's an emergency" as he gently tossed around magazines, stuck tape to magazine pages, and hurriedly and jokingly cut up various pages with a pair of scissors.

Even minor behaviors, if unattended, can have ill effects on the learning climate. For example, Mr. Drake was providing oral instruction pertaining to the use of data his students had collected. A student was tapping his pencil on his table making a drumming noise. Mr. Drake responded mildly to this disruption, "Okay. Let's have our attention up here please." The student stopped tapping for a moment. Mr. Drake replied, "Thank you." All students were quiet and either taking notes, calculating the solution to a problem, or looking at Mr. Drake. Moments later, the student resumed taping his pencil. Mr. Drake did not attend to this and the volume of this student's tapping escalated. Mr. Drake still did not intervene. Rather, he continued to solve another problem with the class, "On paper, I would like to see it set up like this. . . . I would like to see this . . . as the answer." The tapping continued. Some students began to talk. Mr. Drake said, "Okay. I am going to wait until all the talking and all the restlessness ends." The students stopped talking and the one student who was tapping his pencil stopped momentarily. Mr. Drake continued his instruction. One male student then proceeded to grab a calculator from a female student in jest and they had a playful tugging contest. The student who was tapping his pencil began tapping the palm of his hand on the table as well. He created a rhythm with his pencil and hand in combination. He explained to the student next to him, "Look it. If I go with this pen like this, and this hand. . ." and continued his demonstration.

Although sometimes teachers strategically avoid confronting particular students when the behavior is likely to extinguish itself, many maladaptive behaviors, depending on the context of the situation, continue and even escalate, and need an effective intervention. Responding to these incipient behaviors will be described in detail in the indirect and direct interventions sections.

CHAPTER

6

Humor

A student respectfully asked Mr. Elert, "Can I go to sharpen my pencil?" Mr. Elert responded, "I told you you could do it a half hour ago." The student contested, "No. You said I couldn't." Mr. Elert revealed, "I said let the sharpener do it." Several students laughed at this comment. Although Mr. Elert intended the use of humor to be friendly, the student who needed his pencil sharpened did not laugh, smile, nor give any indication that he received the humor well.

Two male students were playfully hitting one another in Mr. Frick's class. Their play escalated to a point that prompted Mr. Frick to respond, "Don't kiss each other." This prompted an insubordinate retort from one of the students, "I'm not using the journal log," referring to a white binder in which students were required to keep their daily journal writing activities. Mr. Frick responded in another lightly sarcastic manner, "You're not using it? You're breakin' my . . ." He then made a pounding motion to his heart with his hands as if to complete the phrase, "You're breaking my heart." Two other students were making shadow figures on the overhead screen. Two others were engaged in physical play trying to grab a pen from one another. Mr. Frick's use of humor to communicate disapproval of the restless behaviors was associated with one student making a mildly challenging comment to Mr. Frick and continued restlessness.

Although humor is often used for the purpose of establishing a rapport or softening a directive to cease a particular behavior, frequently it is misinterpreted and has the opposite effect. For one, humor from an adult is often too sophisticated for young children and adolescents. It can be misinterpreted as humiliating, as humor used in today's media consists largely of demeaning comments. Demeaning humor can readily be accepted by a friend, peer, or family member, but not by a teacher who is formally charged with developing young minds. If a child perceives a classroom teacher as a professional who is responsible for instilling a higher level of moral and academic character, humor that an adult intends to be "witty," can be interpreted as caustic. Secondly, using humor to communicate disapproval of a maladaptive behavior, as some lenient teachers do to avoid direct, assertive communication, often communicates tolerance, or even approval. Humor used to communicate disapproval often serves to reinforce the maladaptive behavior.

Although humor can sometimes be skillfully used to contribute to a positive classroom climate, it is usually not in response to maladaptive behavior. For example, Mr. Gunn was explaining a part of the Cornell note style to a student who was apparently new. He said, "It is a summary in one paragraph of the most important things you learned." The student responded, "So you summarize?" Mr. Gunn asked, "Does that make it easy?" The student answered, "Yeah, I guess." Mr. Gunn added humorously, "And if you have any problems, ask Melissa, she's a professional." Melissa smiled and laughed lightly. Mr. Gunn continued, "She told me that herself." Melissa and the other student both smiled and received the humorous comments well. This seemed to contribute to a more comfortable communication medium between the two girls. The humor appeared to decrease the awkwardness that sometimes accompanies a compliment. Demonstrating humor in a positive manner, not intended to insult, even in jest, is often associated with cooperation, and pleasant interactions.

However, teachers must use humor cautiously. The use of derogatory humor, even in the lightest manner, will not likely contribute to a climate that is characterized by mutual respect. Also, the use of humor to communicate disapproval will often be misinterpreted as approval. Further, students see teachers as a model of expected behavior. If the teacher uses humor too frequently and indiscriminately, frequent and indiscriminate humor will become an accepted behavior among students. Although many do not agree with the teacher adage, "Don't smile until Christmas," if humor is used without discretion, , ironically, teachers need to be prepared to intervene in a disciplinary manner much more frequently.

CHAPTER

7

No Assignment

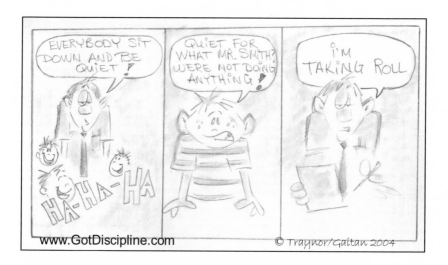

www.GotDiscipline.com   © Traynor/Gaitan 2004

Not having a task for students upon entering Mr. Hannon's classroom seemed to make establishing an effective learning climate more difficult. Prior to the start of his class, several students were laughing and conversing loudly. Despite Mr. Hannon's clear attempt to begin class, "Okay. Let's get seated please," several students continued their conversations. He then intervened by prompting the students to be quiet, "Guys, don't make me count today. You have a test to take and I need you to attempt it." However, the fun-loving atmosphere continued. He followed with another prompt, "Okay. I guess I'm going to have to count."

Not providing students with an activity allows their natural tendency towards disorder to set the learning tone at the beginning of class. Unproductive behaviors range from a few whispers to several casual conversations, teasing, laughing, and horseplay. Such non use of time student time can be contrasted with a practice that provides an assignment for the students upon entering the classroom (see Entering Routines, p. 72)

An analogy to students' apparent natural propensity toward disorder is seen in one of nature's fundamental laws, the law of entropy. Entropy is a measure of the amount of disorder in a system. Nature tends to favor processes that lead to higher entropy or more disorder. The only way to keep or restore order in a system is for the system to expend energy. In a classroom, the amount of effort expended prior to the bell in getting the students to engage in productive behaviors will be well worth the order retained after the bell rings. If keeping students productive at the beginning of the class becomes a consistent practice, the students' conditioning tells them, "Learning occurs from the moment I walk into this classroom." Productive student behaviors at the beginning of class can simply be copying notes from the overhead projector, copying and completing a problem from the board, writing in a journal, or completing a structured reading assignment. Madeleine Hunter labeled these pre-learning exercises sponge activities. Fred Jones (2000) calls them "Bell Work." The purpose of these pre-learning activities is to set a proper learning tone with behaviors consistent with learning, not necessarily to facilitate higher level thought processes. The teacher needs to be free in order to monitor the room and ensure engagement at this crucial moment. The simple tasks mentioned above require little preparation and can be justified as they contribute to a readiness for learning. When the beginning bell rings and the students are

all seated with the proper attitude, they will be ready for
learning.

CHAPTER

8   **Non-Monitoring**

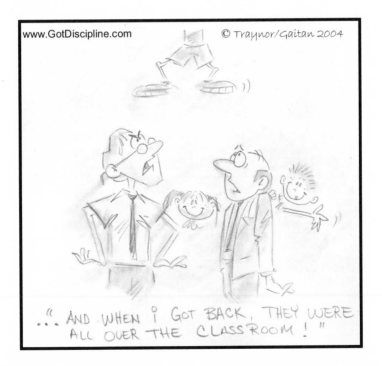

fter the students completed their stretching exercises in
Mr. Incle's PE class, Mr. Incle directed the students to
proceed to the track to begin their timed run, " . . . You

have three minutes . . ." The group of students began to walk
through the basketball courts on their way to the track. Mr.
Incle lagged behind. One boy pushed a friend in jest. An
enthusiastic young man threw a small pebble or at least
pretended to throw one with great force. Three girls were
stayed separate and six boys were horseplaying.

Mr. Jake was walking among the students who were in
turn engaged in an independent textbook assignment. He
proceeded to his desk, sat down, and began to make a phone
call. He said to the person who answered his call, "My name is
Roger Jake. I am a teacher at East Middle School. I'd like to
bring 50 students . . . Alright." He waited, apparently on hold.
Three students began looking around the room at one another
asking questions. Two students were whispering, "Cross this
out . . ." A student in the front was apparently copying another
person's paper. Another student began to whisper. Other
students began to look at others' papers. Although the student
fidgetiness was subtle, Mr. Jake was not satisfied. Upon
concluding his telephone conversation, "Thank you very much.
Bye," he immediately proceeded to a student and asked, "You
okay?" He went to another student and interacted with him,
apparently providing feedback. He proceeded to another student
and asked, "How you doing?" The student replied, "Hard." Mr.
Jake looked closer at his work and asked, "Why did you skip
Section I?" When Mr. Jake returned to walking among the
students, the conversations and movement decreased
tremendously.

The absence of teacher monitoring is associated with
classroom disorder. Sitting at the teacher's desk doing
paperwork, using the computer, gathering information from the
Internet, or preparing lessons are all tempting activities while
students are working productively. However, monitoring, an
indirect intervention described later, is one of the most
powerful, yet simple, interventions available. To determine if
more monitoring is needed, the next few times when attending
to maladaptive behavior, a teacher should reflectively ask, "Was

I sitting at my desk at the time of the incident?" If the answer is frequently affirmative, more frequent monitoring will probably enhance the learning environment.

CHAPTER

9   **General Directives**

Approximately one minute prior to the dismissal bell, Mr. Kettle noticed several small pieces of paper on the floor. Instead of issuing a specific directive such as, "Everyone pick up two pieces of trash," Mr. Kettle announced, "Okay I am excusing you from your seats. So, . . . I am looking for clean floors." One student asked, "It's not clean?" Mr. Kettle attempted to clarify, "Cleaner." Another student questioned, "Cleaner?" Mr. Kettle walked to the back of the room as if to inspect the floor. One student was out of his seat. Instead of directing the student, "Sit down," Mr. Kettle responded in a general manner, "Are you in your seat? Well when you are in your seat . . . " A student exclaimed, "Bell! Alright! Come on!" The students then left.

During another period Mr. Kettle was explaining an assignment using the overhead projector. A student blurted, "We don't have school on Friday, do we?" Several students began talking. Instead of directing the students specifically to stop talking, Mr. Kettle responded, "Guess what? No learning is talking place right now." Several students quieted momentarily but then began conversing again. Another student called out, "We did this yesterday." During the assignment, several students began conversing again. Mr. Kettle intervened in another general manner, "You know the quality of your writing decreases when you are talking." However, the students continued talking.

Providing a general as opposed to specific directive for students to stop conversing, clean the room, or sit in their seats is associated with non-compliance. General directives communicate that following the directive is optional and punishment unlikely. For example, Mr. Kettle's general directive for students to be quiet, "Guess what? No learning is talking place right now," did not communicate clearly enough to the talking students to cease. This is consistent with Brint (1998), "Without great clarity and much repetition, shadows are likely to fall between the expression of teachers and the interpretations of those expressions by students" (p. 261). Providing explicit directives, described later, provides a nice contrast to this ineffective practice.

CHAPTER

10   Reinforcing Callouts

While making preliminary announcements, Mr. Leonard commented in frustration, "This is the most talkative class." This seemed to elicit a spontaneous question from a student, "That's bad huh?" Instead of directing the class to quit talking or raise their hands prior to asking a question, Mr. Leonard answered the student, "No. It's not bad, it's social." Mr. Leonard proceeded with his announcements amid several conversations and noted a lack of glue sticks for the students' projects, "We are running out of glue sticks I'm afraid." Again a student freely called out, "Can I go out and get some?" and again, Mr. Leonard responded, "No. We'll just use tape." The cycle of students calling out, addressing the teacher at will, and the teacher responding to the callouts continued through the end of Mr. Leonard's explanation. After several cycles, only a few students remained attentive. One student yelled from the back of the room, "Mr. Leonard!"

Following an established procedure for addressing the teacher, such as traditional hand-raising, is a common practice in many effective classrooms. Although highly effective, this procedure requires effort to establish and must consistently be reinforced. Freely asking the teacher a question is quite natural to an untrained student as is responding to the question. In informal settings where no real learning objectives exist, one-on-one dialogues are entirely appropriate. However, when bringing an entire class toward mastery of a specific learning objective is the goal, having a procedure for addressing the teacher, such as hand-raising, will increase efficiency and effectiveness immensely. If a student calls out, the teacher should avoid the natural temptation to answer and simply refer the student to the established procedure. If students feel free to call out at any moment, they tend to interrupt the teacher and other students. A teacher can enforce hand-raising by acknowledging students who raise their hands but still not allow them to call out. Following are two illustrations that show how this procedure contributes to the maintenance of a productive learning environment.

Ms. Michael's students had completed their reading aloud phonics exercise and returned to their seats. She was beginning to provide further direction to her class when a student raised her hand. Ms. Michael responded, "One minute, Baby," and continued with her directions. The student cooperatively lowered her hand. Apparently the student answered her own question, as she did not raise her hand again.

Mr. Noako directed the students to work on their projects in groups. A student raised his hand and Mr. Noako promptly said, "I'll be right with you, Johnny." The student replied, "Okay," and he waited patiently. Moments later Mr. Naoko attended to the student, who in turn, responded politely.

Some teachers counter that not having a procedure for addressing a teacher permits productive interaction. For example, Mr. Orosco was engaging the students in a discussion pertaining to the ethnicities of people of Spanish speaking countries. A student freely asked, "What about Peru?" Mr. Orosco reinforced the student response, "Peru," and continued with an explanation, " . . . and a person from Peru is Peruvian." Another student enthusiastically called out a response pertaining to France. Mr. Orosco reinforced this response by asking the students, "Francés is what language?" Another student immediately responded, "French." Mr. Orosco positively reinforced this student's answer by saying, "That is a really excellent guess because it sounds like . . ." and he continued the free interaction with his students.

Although frequently creating this open dialogue forum can be productive, a teacher must be cautious. Teachers who do not establish a hand-raising procedure or the like, must stay alert and be prepared to intervene toward attending to frequent side conversations that will certainly erupt.

CHAPTER

11   **End of Class**

Toward the end of the period, Mr. Phi's directive for the students to complete their worksheet, "Let's finish them up," appeared to prompt several students to rise from their seats. Two others were so disengaged that they did not realize Mr. Phi was collecting calculators from them. Mr. Phi's final announcements began with, "Alright ladies and gentlemen, before you go, I have a reminder . . . " and seemed to communicate to eight other students that the class was over, as they also rose from their seats.

Referring to the period nearing completion triggers the conditioned dismissal responses students have learned and provides a safe opportunity for students to communicate nonverbally to the teacher their desire to leave. Ignoring the dismissal behaviors of students further provides tacit approval for students to continue to gather their materials and disengage from learning. Teachers should avoid inadvertently referring to the end of the period.

CATEGORY **2** –

NURTURING PRACTICES

Nurturing practices are characterized by concern, respect, and caring. Young (1993) expresses the need to develop a positive, trusting relationship with a challenging child as a first step in a strategy for positively influencing behavior and development. Young argues that because many students' home environments are unpredictable, they need exposure to caring adults who value them and who establish school settings that are consistent, predictable, and supportive. Engelmann and Colvin (1983) point out that teacher and student interactions could be positive or negative depending on whether the teacher is responding to appropriate or inappropriate behavior. They suggest that at least 80% of all interactions should be positive.

The nurturing practices are in the left middle of the continuum model in Figure 1. As shown, they are readily available to the lenient and moderate teachers. Although these practices are listed as effective, the nurturing practices without the other interventions will not produce an entirely effective learning environment. A synergistic relationship appears to exist between nurturing practices and direct interventions. If behaviors consistent with learning are well established, the nurturing practices add a positive learning tone to the room characterized by a climate of respect and caring far greater than if nurturing practices were implemented alone. Behaviors consistent with learning must be established in order for the nurturing practices to have their optimal effect. This is consistent with DeMarrais and LeCompte (1999), "Teachers maintain control only by balancing personal forcefulness with intimate teacher-pupil relationships" (p. 169).

As illustrated in Figure 1, a teacher strongly identified with the lenient approach, does not have the direct interventions readily available. The following episode is from an observation of a teacher strongly identified with the lenient approach. It illustrates the effects of too great an emphasis on nurturing practices over direct interventions.

An orderly environment was perhaps not as important to Mr. Quail as maintaining relationships with students. Mr. Quail was having difficulty making some final announcements prior to dismissing the class. He raised his hand to draw attention to himself and announced, "One last thing we . . . Actually two last things. No. Three last things." Several students were still inattentive, a few still conversing. Mr. Quail responded to the state of the classroom in disappointment, "You are so talkative." He continued, "One, you have a homework assignment." He pointed to the white board with the homework assignment written on it and provided a brief explanation. He continued, "Two, I am not going to be here on Monday. Mr. Edwards, I think, will be here." A student exclaimed joyfully, "Yeah!" Mr. Quail continued, "I expect good behavior. And three, the most important thing, have a nice day." No bell was heard, but the students left at the close of this announcement. Mr. Quail's last statement appeared to suggest having "a nice day" was more important to him than the students demonstrating "good behavior" consistent with learning.

Teachers strongly identified with the lenient approach should not abandon their nurturing practices. However, the nurturing practices will be much more effective in contributing to a respectful climate, if the behaviors consistent with learning are concomitantly established.

CHAPTER

12   Greetings

Mr. Urea was participating in light conversations and greeting students at the door as they entered prior to the beginning of class. He enthusiastically greeted one boy, "Hello Ismael," and another girl, "Flor, how are you today?" He graciously inquired to another, "How are you today?" and commented to someone else, "Looking good. Did you bring your work today?" He then politely announced to group of 10 students around the door, "It's about time to close. Better get in." The students respectfully entered. He said to the final student entering, "Real long line at Snack?" The student walked up with a small beanbag type ball called a Hacky Sac. Mr. Urea responded as if to communicate interest, "Hacky Sac." The student grinned and entered. The students were taking their seats, many conversing in a civilized manner.

Greeting students at the entrance door, provides a low risk opportunity for teachers to set a tone of courtesy and professionalism. This practice communicates teacher interest in each student. An added advantage is that inappropriate behaviors can be halted at the door. Occasionally, students enter the classroom demonstrating behaviors that are tolerated outdoors, but entirely inappropriate indoors. A teacher at the entrance door has the opportunity to privately intervene to subdue any behaviors not consistent with learning. Mere proximity to the child can suppress maladaptive behavior. One teacher summarized this effective practice, "It calms them down. When they come in, some have high energy. It allows me to make contact with each one. And sometimes I just stand outside if it is noisy. It's kind of like 'big brother is watching.'"

CHAPTER

13 Modeling Respect

One student entered Mr. Vick's class late while the others were engaged in an exam. Mr. Vick questioned the student who apparently had no pass or verification for being unsupervised outside of the classroom. Mr. Vick questioned, "Were you on time out?" The student, upon closer examination, had a bag of ice and paper towel over his hand. He was apparently injured from a fall or an accident from a physical activity. Upon observing this, Mr. Vick demonstrated concern and asked in a caring tone, "What happened?" The student remained quiet. He proceeded to gather materials and instructions for the student without further questioning. Absent from this interaction was a reprimanding tone that might normally prevail when a student enters late. Mr. Vick did not send the student back to get a pass for being late, he did not issue the student a reprimanding consequence either. The consequences for being tardy were overlooked due to the genuine concern Mr. Vick had for the student. He was able to demonstrate the respect through showing concern and actually gathering materials the student needed. The rest of the students also remained engaged in the exam undisturbed by the interaction.

Demonstrating concern or good manners is associated with maintenance of respect in the classroom. The teacher in the classroom is the professional and should strive to model a professional demeanor at all times. This sometimes means being flexible and using genuine student concern to guide actions rather than rigid rules. Having a climate of mutual respect is clearly impossible if the teacher does not demonstrate respect toward students. Although being firm and implementing direct, explicit interventions might be necessary, if a teacher has established behaviors consistent with learning as the norm, demonstrating respect toward students should be done at every opportunity.

CHAPTER

14 Appropriate Responses

Mrs. Xyland was providing oral instruction on reading a passage with different tones of voice. She queried a boy named Kyle, who was slouching in the front row. He responded, "What?" revealing that he was not attentive. Mrs. Xyland responded non-confrontationally, "I wasn't trying to trick you. I thought you knew the answer." Mrs. Xyland asked the class another question. Kyle raised his hand to respond indicating that he was now attentive and willing to participate. Mrs. Xyland's preservation of Kyle's dignity by avoiding public admonishment was observed to be associated with Kyle's productive participation moments later.

Responses to inappropriate behavior that demonstrate teacher restraint and politeness are associated with maintenance of order, student preservation of dignity, compliance, and continued engagement in instruction.

CATEGORY **3** –

INDIRECT PRACTICES

W alker, Colvin, and Ramsey (1995) put forth that private teacher responses, gentle reminders of agreed upon behaviors, and interacting with students in non-confrontational ways using polite redirecting comments, serve a teacher well toward maintaining appropriate classroom order (p. 75-76). Why confront a student directly when an indirect intervention will do? According to Figure 1, the indirect interventions appear accessible to all teachers regardless of how strongly they are identified with a particular approach. They are also quite effective. Although these practices require a combination of skill, preparation, or good judgment, the well-developed fortitude of a veteran is not needed.

CHAPTER

15 High Accountability

Ms. Zimmer checked each student's reading log progress and asked questions such as "Do you have your reading log, Hun?" The students then showed Ms. Zimmer their reading logs. Ms. Zimmer routinely recorded students' independent reading and the students generally reported to her their progress. She also collected writing entries from students apparently on a weekly basis and the students diligently participated in their independent daily writing exercises.

Mr. Abraham' class was engaged in an independent assignment when he called a student to his desk. This student was engaged in an off-task conversation with another student earlier. Mr. Abraham had a computer printout ready, pointed to a score, and said, "That's nice. But some of these are not as nice. I want you to . . . If you keep pumping these hundreds in there . . ." The student listened attentively. The student brought the printout back to his desk and shared his record with another student. He appeared interested in this set of data and told the other student, "I've got to get my grades up to an A." The discussion and printout of records were associated with a change in the topic of conversation and demeanor for this student. Mr.

Abraham appeared to correctly predict that showing this student actual classroom progress would prompt him to become more serious.

Monitoring student progress maintains motivation. Although teacher enthusiasm and intrinsically interesting assignments will increase motivation, students often do not comprehend the long-term benefits of mastering unappealing material. Brooks (1985) amplifies this point, "If you believe that learning should be fun, you are doing the students a disservice. The student becomes a victim, thinking that everything in life should be fun" (p.76). A student will know a teacher values particular assignments if the teacher routinely provides quick, objective, and understandable feedback. Children need to know with points, percentages, gold stars, etc., that their work has value.

CHAPTER

16 Monitoring

Ms. Bradford disclosed that her student desks were arranged for the purpose of being able to monitor students by walking among them, "I have a variation on the basic U shape. I can get to any kid at any time in a handful of seconds." Her arrangement of student desks provided her with this immediate access (Figure 2). Toward the back of the room, facing the dry erase board, were two columns, each with four desks. Between the dry erase board and this group of eight desks were two groups of desks on the opposite sides of the room facing the center of the class. These groups consisted of four columns and three rows of desks for a total of 12 on each side. The short depth of the columns, three rows deep on the sides of the room, and the back center location of the two columns of four rows, provided quick access to students and teacher visibility. For example, even if Ms. Bradford was helping students in one of the back desks along the side wall, she would still be seen by all students and could certainly "get to any kid . . . in a handful of seconds."

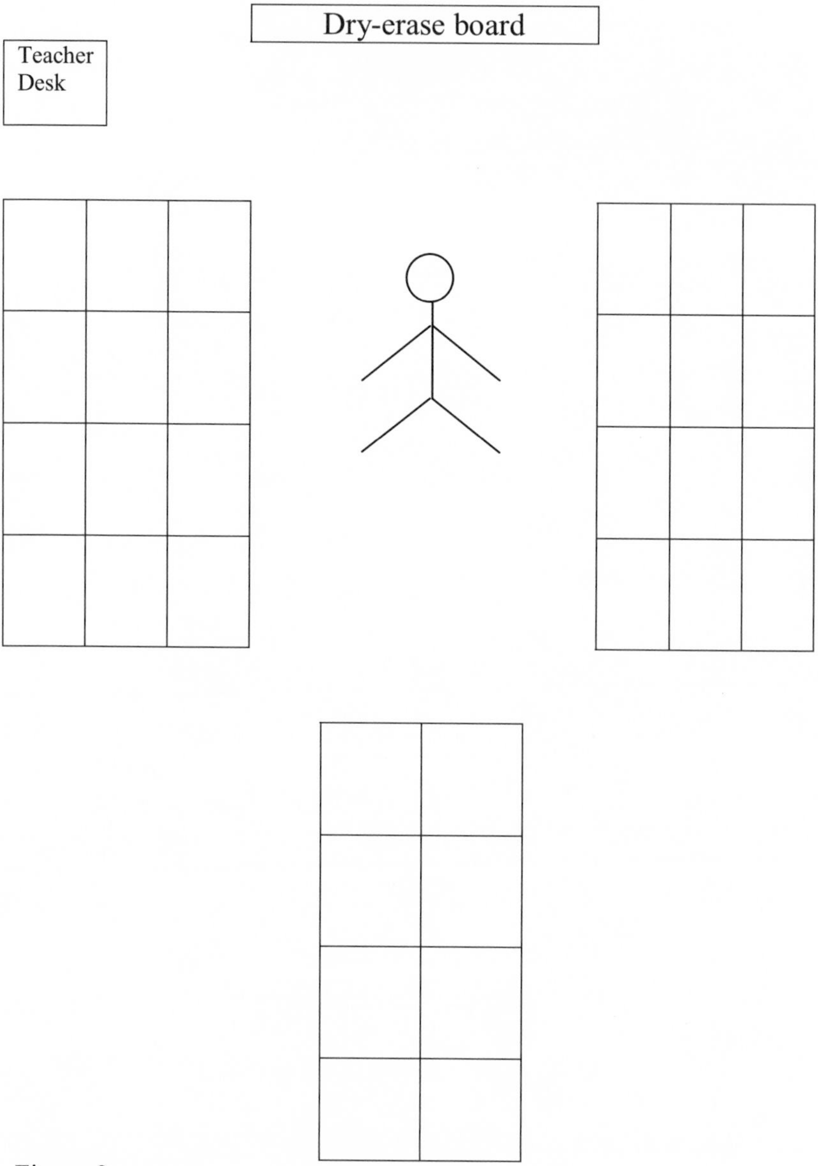

Dry-erase board

Teacher Desk

Figure 2
Variation of Desks in a Basic "U" Shape.
Note: Arranged for student and teacher proximity. Each square represents one desk.

Ms. Bradford was walking among students with her clipboard, collecting reading log scores. She commented to one student, "Thank you for showing . . . Good job." She crouched down to another student and asked, "Alexandria? Can you hand this out?" She asked another student, "Reading log?" The student turned over her paper. Ms. Bradford replied, "Good." She continued walking among the students, collecting their reading log scores, and the students continued writing independently. She was able to interact efficiently and effectively with every student.

As stated in the non-monitoring section, monitoring is perhaps the most powerful proactive classroom management strategy. A strong teacher presence made known by walking among students suppresses the students' natural propensity toward disorder. Another effective teacher emphasizes:

A lot of it is walking around. Proximity is important. Proximity is the most important thing in control. You got to be looking at their work. I can't be sitting here at the desk and they are doing something brand new or very difficult or at the outside edge of their ability. I can't sit back here. I've got to be walking up and down making sure everybody's doing the right thing – that nobody's lost.

CHAPTER

17   **Implicit Interactions**

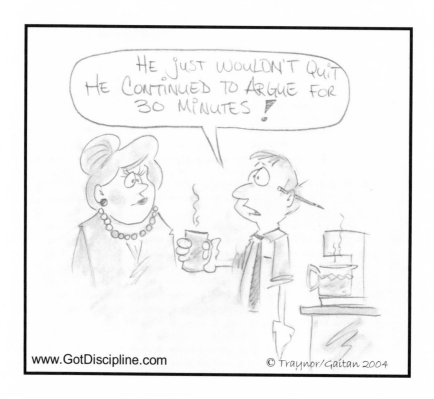

Taking a student and teacher quarrel out of the spectacle for all to observe often removes from the student the motivation necessary for continued confrontation. To a child, how a teacher perceives him or her is insignificant compared to peer-perception. This is especially true for older students. Some students continue arguing simply because they know their peers are watching and do not want to be perceived as forfeiting the argument. Frequently, teachers communicate overtly to prompt students to refocus when more subtle communication would be more effective.

✱ ✱ ✱

Private Interactions

A student entered Mr. Clavel's classroom late while the class was engaged in an exam. Mr. Clavel whispered a question to the student privately. The student responded at first a bit agitated, "I don't know, I don't know!" Mr. Clavel then whispered again to the student. The student stopped talking and joined the class.

Private as opposed to public directives remove individual student and teacher interaction from classroom focus and therefore does not disrupt instruction. If intervention is required to suppress a maladaptive behavior, private interaction is far more likely to de-escalate the behavior than public interaction. Private interaction avoids public embarrassment and therefore does not necessitate student defensive responses.

Apart from any defensive motives, students frequently call for teacher attention as part of the normal instructional process. If students are focused independently, teacher interaction with an individual has the potential to disrupt an otherwise pleasant classroom learning tone. For example, interacting with a student from across the room not only draws unnecessary attention from individuals engaged in their lesson, such a disruption tends to induce side talking. A teacher can use private interaction to maintain the learning tone. Walking over to a student with a raised hand as opposed to calling on the student from across the room will likely leave the classroom climate undisturbed.

✳ ✳ ✳

Strategic Avoidance

Students in Mr. Duarte's Spanish class were rehearsing dialogues in pairs. As they became ready, they volunteered to perform before the class. One student, Derrick, entered the room while one pair of students was concluding their performance to an attentive class. Mr. Duarte said, "Muy bien," signifying his approval of the performing pair. Derrick then announced rather blatantly, "I'm ready." He seemed to get no reinforcement for this call out from other students. Derrick told his partner in the same volume and tone, as if he wished the entire class to hear, "Sorry to put you through this, I know you might not be ready." Derrick then began to read his part of the dialogue. However, the other student did not respond. Derrick, with his same loud tone continued, "Say, 'Hola y tu?' Okay? I know you don't know Spanish, but you have to read." Awkward silence permeated the room as Derrick appeared to expect recognition from his classmates or at least a reprimand from Mr. Duarte for his overt behavior. Neither came, and the class continued rehearsing their dialogues.

Although a teacher should not simply ignore all maladaptive behaviors, strategically avoiding some types of confrontations can allow the behavior to cease on its own. The teacher must decide whether intervention or non-intervention will de-escalate the behavior more. If non-intervention is the choice, a follow-up private interaction can have a positive impact.

✳ ✳ ✳

Waiting

The students in Miss Eagle's remedial language arts class were engaged in their routine independent writing assignment at the beginning of the period. While Miss Eagle walked among them with her clipboard, collecting reading log scores, she began to announce, "When you score . . ." However, some students were not attentive, so she stopped. Miss Eagle paused for a moment and said, "Good," as the class quieted. She continued, "When you score . . ." and she paused again, gazing around the room, as some students tried to continue with their previous conversations. The class quieted even more in response to this pause. She continued, "Please score your reading log and your warm ups." By then, all students were fully attentive.

Later in the period, Miss Eagle orally reviewed nouns with the class. She used "socks" as an example and asked, "Can you smell, see, hear, taste, touch . . ." Several students together said, "Yes." A student commented that socks could not be heard. Miss. Eagle explained that slapping the socks against something could produce sound. Several students laughed in response. She continued, "If you can smell, see, hear, taste, touch. . . If you can do any of these, then it is a noun. If you can think about them, . . . abstract nouns." She then continued with instruction but a few students began talking. Miss Eagle stood abruptly, placed her hands at her sides as if to communicate that she was waiting. One student exclaimed, "Shut up, people!" The students again became silent.

Conspicuously waiting for student attention can stop restless behaviors. This intervention is often more effective than directly telling a student to be quiet. One frequent student response to a teacher directive to be quiet is, "But I wasn't talking." Simply waiting for a student or a group of students to stop talking can clearly communicate the same message. Responding, "I was not talking," to a teacher who has not explicitly accused anyone of talking would be rather awkward.

The Cub Scout organization is well known for having a signal, a two finger peace sign, that all scouts know means to be quiet. When a scout leader displays this "peace sign," no scouts ever say, "We weren't talking," as they have not been accused of talking. The message is simply, "It is now time to be quiet."

❋ ❋ ❋

Body Language

Mr. Fogherty was explaining the procedure for the students' journal entries and was writing on the board. He explained, "You have a choice, three journal topics. . . . So it will be a thesis. Your thesis will be the last statement before . . ." He was writing onto the dry erase board a summary of the main points he wished to convey. His back was to the class. Two students began conversing. Mr. Fogherty swiftly turned and focused directly and sternly on the pair. The students then immediately stopped talking.

The students in Ms. Garret's class were engaged in independent writing. Ms. Garret sat erect at her desk, looking at her computer screen and students intermittently. One student rose and began to change seats. Ms. Garret turned her head, spotted the student, and the student returned to her original seat. Another student began giggling. Ms. Garret abruptly stared at this student. The student stopped giggling but did not reengage in writing. Ms. Garret did not unlock her stare. Another student innocently asked Ms. Garret permission to work on another assignment, "Ms. Garret, can we work on . . .?" Ms. Garret nodded her head affirmatively but still did not unlock her stare from the student who was previously giggling. The student began to giggle again, but apparently knowing that Ms. Garret was watching, did not continue. The rest of the class remained engaged as if unconcerned with the giggling student. The student began to speak to Ms. Garret, but Ms. Garret sharply interrupted, "Don't talk to me." The student proceeded to work immediately and Ms. Garret then unlocked her stare. The student continued writing.

Diaz-Rico and Weed (2002), in their description of nonverbal communication assert, "Body language is one way in which teachers communicate their authority in the classroom" (p. 68). Purposeful movements accompanied by intent looks are powerful ways to communicate disapproval of maladaptive behavior. Again, the teacher has provided nothing overt against which to ague and thereby avoids drawing attention to the interaction. Arguing against silence is too awkward for students. Peers are more likely to think the student is odd for responding to no directive than if the student was responding to an explicit directive. Using silent, implicit directives also have the advantage of not disturbing the rest of the class and not drawing an audience to the student.

✻ ✻ ✻

Continuing with Instruction

Mr. Haskel was asking his students Spanish terminology questions, "What's baja?" A student answered in a joking tone, "Bajamas," and a few students began to laugh. Mr. Haskel responded, "Good," and continued with an explanation of how baja means low and can be used in geography. He provided another example of Baja California meaning below California. The laughter stopped as he continued his instruction. During the same part of the lesson, Mr. Haskel questioned, "What do we normally call Chile?" A student called out, "Beans and meat," in a similar joking tone of voice. This again appeared to elicit laughter from the students and Mr. Haskel again quickly, and politely interrupted, "Yeah. Normally we refer to beans," and immediately continued, "What else do we think of?" A student responded, "Hot." Mr. Haskel responded, "Yes, we actually think about peppers." He then continued with an explanation of the country, Chile, and how it got its name. The laughter did not continue through Mr. Haskel's instruction.

Skillfully continuing with instruction during moments where a direct confrontation would risk compromising the classroom climate is often associated with a de-escalation of unproductive behavior. This is a technique used by comedians on the stage with hecklers. The comedian is in control of the microphone and will only continue banter with a heckler if it serves the comedian's own purpose. If the banter is no longer productive, the comedian will move on and continue with his spiel. Retaining control of the presentation is usually better than trying to control the disruption or disruptor.

Judgment and expertise are important for this intervention. A teacher must exercise good judgment and not ignore maladaptive behaviors that are likely to escalate as in the avoidance section. Also, being an expert in the content of the presentation gives the teacher much more control. As in the above example, Mr. Haskel, being a master of his content, was able to redirect the disruptions by referring to his lesson's content. Also, if the presentation component of a lesson is well structured, simply refocusing on the structured presentation will more likely put the teacher back in authority.

❋ ❋ ❋

Gestures

Mr. Island held up his open hand, palm outward, to one student who was about to interrupt his conversation with another student. This appeared to nonverbally and non-argumentatively communicate a clear directive to not interrupt. Later, Mr. Island held a finger to his lips to communicate to a student who was intending to freely ask a question. This was during the time the others were engaged in their independent writing assignment. Again, Mr. Island's silent gesture did not disturb the class and did not provide the student the opportunity to call out. Pointing to a student's desk in reaction to a student who was approaching him also clearly communicated to the student to return to his seat. The pointing further did not disrupt the class and did not provide an appropriate medium for a response.

Mr. Island's non-verbal gestures communicated specifically and privately to individuals. Like body language and conspicuously waiting, gestures that imply commands are associated with compliance, as they too do not provide a public medium in which to argue.

CHAPTER

18   **Preparation**

No classroom management practice will be effective without sufficient preparation. Gettinger (1988) states that quality instruction is one of the most fundamental proactive classroom management strategies. Walker, Colvin, and Ramsey (1995) add that fewer problems occur when students are fully engaged academically (p. 161). In addition to instructional preparation, other preparations can contribute substantially toward building a productive environment.

✹ ✹ ✹

Inviting Environment

Mrs. Jacob's classroom was set up to create a comfortable inviting atmosphere. In the back corner of the classroom opposite the entrance door was a couch with two pillows. In front of the couch was a circular card table. Along the back wall was a broom with the bristles arranged in a circular manner like a witch's broom. To the right of the entrance door was a large seven-foot cabinet with an alphabet poster on it. Another poster was titled, "How are you feeling today?" with pictures of 30 faces of various expressions, each described by words such as angry, tired, bored, happy, etc. Apparently knowing how her students felt was important to Mrs. Jacob. Her arrangement of desks also provided ample space in the center of the room in which students could gather for various activities.

Mrs. Jacob was reading to her students in a dynamic voice while sitting in a white wicker chair in the front of the room. All students were listening attentively. Ten were lying down comfortably in the center. Fifteen were sitting in the desks along the perimeter. A female student was sitting comfortably in Mrs. Jacob's teacher chair, which was away from her desk for this reading activity. The classroom climate, with the students comfortably lying on the floor or sitting, relaxed at their desks being read to in a caring, enthusiastic manner, appeared similar to the emotional climate that exists when a parent reads a bedtime story to a child.

A student commenting, "It's nice in here," upon entering the room is pleasant to hear and certainly gives the teacher an advantage toward building a respectful climate. Although preparing the physical environment in an inviting manner takes an artistic talent and effort similar to an interior decorator, efforts toward this end will certainly not have any negative effects. Additionally, once the physical environment is prepared, it does not need attention during the critical moments – when the children are present.

❋ ❋ ❋

Materials

Mr. Kastle had gathered several materials and placed them on a front center table for students to use for their project. The materials included magazines, scissors, rulers, colored pencils, and extra paper. During the lesson, students readily gathered their materials and brought them back to their work stations. No time was wasted waiting for materials, assigning tasks of gathering and distributing materials, or waiting for the teacher to distribute materials to each work station. Students made no complaints regarding being given an extra paper or not being given a colored pencil, etc., either.

A student approached Mr. Long and asked him for the assignments for the next few days, as he was planning on being absent. Mr. Long first responded with a disappointed tone, "I really have not got that up yet." However, he appeared to suddenly realize that he had a worksheet prepared that was underneath the dry erase board's cupboard a few feet away. He said, "Well, one thing right here," retrieved the worksheet from the cupboard, and handed it to the student. Having his assignments prepared in a readily accessible area was associated with this student having access to and being provided with genuine classroom instructional material during his absence. Mr. Long did not need to excuse this student from this assignment or have the student complete the assignment upon his return.

Teacher preparation and distribution of materials at key locations in the classroom facilitates student access. Preparing materials prior to class and knowing where to access them will only contribute to more organization and order in a classroom. In contrast, not having necessary materials prepared can be quite debilitating to a teacher charged with the responsibility of keeping students orderly. Teacher time is valuable in every classroom session and everything practically possible should be done prior to the start of class to preserve this time.

❊ ❊ ❊

Visual Aides

Mr. Mango was explaining how different words are used in different languages to describe animal sounds. As Mr. Mango was providing oral examples of these words, such as "pio," in French, for the sound a chick makes, and "meow," in English, for the sound a cat makes, several students began laughing. Although this laughter was not made in disrespect or defiance of Mr. Mango, it was not productive. Further, continuing with this activity appeared likely to escalate the laughter. However, Mr. Mango subtly, yet quickly, transitioned from this lesson. Prior to class, he had written on chart paper attached to an easel, a Spanish song, "Frey Felipe" sung to the tune of, "Are You Sleeping?" The easel faced the students at the front of the room. The print was sufficiently large for all students to read without straining. After he provided the last animal sound example, he said, "Repeat" and pointed to the print on the easel, "Frey Felipe." The students, without hesitation and without carrying over any laughter repeated in unison, "Frey Felipe."

During a poster building activity in Mr. Nguyen's science class, one student appeared a bit frustrated. He walked to the front of the room and picked up a paper with directions. He returned to his table and opened his backpack. He disclosed to another student, "I'm going to get in trouble by my dad." Mr. Nguyen turned to this student and asked, "Where's your work?" The student apparently did not understand what to do and would require a long re-orientation if he were to successfully complete the poster. However, Mr. Nguyen had prepared a drawing on the dry erase board, a model of the atom the students were to construct. It had proton and neutron representations on it. Mr. Nguyen referred to this illustration adding, "Come here, this is a model." He pointed to the protons and asked the student, "How many protons?" Similarly he pointed to the neutrons and asked, "How many neutrons?" The student responded readily, looking at the model during his explanation.

Simple diagrams, models, or other visual aides can reinforce learning. Knowing that these visual aides will provide more focus on or understanding of the learning objective, a prudent teacher will prepare them prior to the lesson. If students are focused on learning, they are likely demonstrating the behaviors consistent with learning. Preparing anything prior to the lesson that will focus the students' attention on learning will serve a teacher well in managing behaviors.

❊ ❊ ❊

Physical Environment

Ms. Oscar used the space she created in the center of her
classroom for student gathering during their phonics routines.
She briefly reviewed the procedure for gathering and then
counted down from nine, "nine, eighth, seven, . . ." The students
efficiently left their seats, proceeded to the center of the room,
and waited before the count of one. They repeated sounds and
followed instructions. For example, Ms. Oscar demonstrated,
"Say 'Rag.'" The students then responded, "Rag." Ms. Oscar
repeated herself to follow an even rhythm, "Say 'Rag.'" The
students again repeated within the rhythm, "Rag." Ms. Oscar
continued within the rhythm, "Say 'Rag' without the /g/ sound."
The students then made the sound, "Răˇ." Ms. Oscar was
apparently following a script with a distinct rhythm, and the
students, altogether in the space created in the center of the
room, recited, as in a chorus.

Mr. Peter's PE students were standing on the blacktop,
conversing, and waiting for the class to begin. After he emerged
from the locker room and blew his whistle, four students
returned their basketballs to the metal cart. His students
promptly sat inside numbered painted squares as they became
ready for their attendance warm up activities. Preparing
designated locations for student activities is associated with
compliance.

The physical environment can be manipulated to
accommodate student movement and activities. Anthropology
has long held that the physical setting has much to do with
affecting and shaping human behavior. When entering a
classroom, a student immediately knows where teacher
instruction occurs, where to sit, where pencils get sharpened,
where materials are distributed, or where experiments are
performed by virtue of how the room is arranged. Student desk
arrangement can encourage student-student interactions,

student-teacher interaction, or even thwart interactions. Efforts toward manipulating the physical environment toward managing student behavior prior to student arrival decreases the need to manage behavior after the students arrive. For example, if having students gather in key areas for specific activities is part of the teacher's plan, preparing these areas prior to instruction will serve to guide student behavior during the activity. If independent work on an exam is desired, arranging desks with ample space between them would promote independent engagement.

❊ ❊ ❊

Professional Dress

Many teachers recognize a significant increase in student respect if they dress professionally. Some have even said that it enhances their own professional demeanor. If this is true, the extra cost in clothes is well worth it. Professional dress also has the added benefit of making a professional impression on parents. Student respect is far more easily obtained if the parents respect the teacher as a professional. Parents subconsciously communicate attitudes about their child's teacher to their child. Not having parental respect creates great barriers toward gaining student respect.

Although dressing less professionally will not necessarily evoke poor behavior and poor parental support, if a parent raises concerns about a teacher to the principal, and the teacher in question does not dress professionally, the parent may also express concern about dress to support their case of a teacher's general ineffectiveness. Sloppy dress reinforces students' and parents' negative assumptions about a teacher.

Frequently, teachers believe that dressing down to the students' level decreases barriers to a genuine relationship. However, a relationship without professional respect will do little toward instilling behaviors consistent with mastery of a rigorous curriculum. Dressing professionally is a strategy that is relatively easy to implement. One caution, teachers should not sacrifice too much comfort when selecting shoes. Effective teachers walk among students frequently throughout the day and should take great care of their feet.

CATEGORY **4** –

DIRECT PRACTICES

E ffective teachers use direct practices to explicitly and assertively guide student behavior. Consequences for misbehavior are used as a deterrent and are intended specifically not to harm the students' physical or emotional state of being. Gaddy and Kelly (1984), in their description of strategies for creating a safe school climate suggest that firm, fair, and sensitive policies are the key components in establishing and maintaining school discipline. They add that fair, quick and consistent, punitive and positive consequences should be judiciously given using due process. Collette and Chiapette (1989) insist this type of enforcement is a positive one that permits teachers to maintain the best possible learning environment in a firm, non-hostile, and constructive way.

Being direct does not suggest using coercion. Student dignity and teacher professionalism must be preserved when implementing these practices. According to Figure 1, teachers strongly identified with the moderate and rigid approach have less difficulty implementing direct interventions.

CHAPTER

19   Behavioral Systems

A student in Miss Quinn's classroom read aloud from the dry erase board the learning for the week. Miss Quinn prompted the students to discuss it, "Okay, that was the learning for the week. Talk to each other." She waited for approximately 20 seconds and continued, "Okay, look up here." However, not all students stopped talking. Miss Quinn responded by counting, "One, two, three." The students then became quiet and attentive. Miss Quinn responded, "Excellent," turned to a student in a front corner seat and said, "That's a minute, Honey." Apparently this student was the record keeper of all of the minutes the class earned or lost.

Students entering Mr. Rodriguez's algebra, class joked with one another, and were a bit noisy. Mr. Rodriguez announced at the beginning, "Let's get to work." However, the students continued their commotion. Mr. Rodriguez then began counting in German. A few students said, "Shhh" and one student's name in particular was declared by another student. All but one student stopped talking. Another student encouraged this student to stop, "Come on!" The remaining student stopped and all were attentive.

The behavior systems used in the above episodes contained a counting procedure with implicit consequences if the students did not behave in accordance with established standards. Normally, administering negative consequences for maladaptive behavior, even if judiciously assigned, evokes emotional conflict. The goal in implementing a system is to reduce the tendency for the conflict to manifest itself in disruptive manners. Referring to and implementing a fair and established behavior system in a consistent manner takes the arbitrary nature away from the punishment. One effective teacher who used Lee Canter's assertive discipline described:

> [If] you have a discipline plan in place and you follow it every time, I find if you put one name on the board, you can quiet a whole class down. Everything just stops. And it's not a threat. I mean I'm just a record keeper.

Fair behavior systems, consistently applied in an equitable manner reveal that the teacher is "just a record keeper," that the consequence was a result of the student's wrong doing, and not at the whim of the teacher.

CHAPTER

20 Explicit Directives

M s. Stanley's students began writing. One student
approached her for an eraser. Ms. Stanley responded,
"You need to sit down right now and when we are
finished, I will give you one." The student immediately
complied. Ms. Stanley then walked to the side of the room.
Two students began to converse and one student rose from his
seat. Ms. Stanley directed, "Sit down and start to write." The
student complied and the class remained engaged. Ms. Stanley
then proceeded to record scores. She called one student's name
asking, "How many lines?" The student responded, "Fourteen."
She then addressed the class as she noticed a few students
conversing, "Okay, friends . . . Silent . . . Silent." The class
became silent. Moments later, one student became ambulatory.
Ms. Stanley responded, "Sit." However, the student contested
by explaining the rationale for being out of his seat. Ms.
Stanley repeated, "Sit, sit," and the student complied.

Clear, explicit directives can be effective when used
skillfully at the right moment. Defying a clear, unequivocal
directive can only be interpreted as insubordination, too great a
risk for most students. A skillful teacher, like a skillful chess
player, sees a few "moves" ahead and is able to warn the student

with a reasonable consequence that will leave a productive climate in tact. Generally, if a student defies a teacher's clear directive, an effective teacher will warn the student of an impending consequence for continued defiance and efficiently administer the consequence in a professional manner as necessary. Follow through after a warning of a phone call home is one of the most effective consequences a teacher can provide. Phone calls home are discussed in a later section.

Maintaining professionalism is absolutely essential regardless of what behaviors the student demonstrates. Testing a teacher's willingness to implement consequences is in the nature of a classroom. Arguing with a student has seldom resulted in productive acquiescence to the teacher's reasoning. However, if consequences are fair, consistent, and equitably applied, students will stop testing the teacher's authority and student compliance will become established as the norm.

CHAPTER

21   Routines

When routines serve an instructional purpose, establishing them in the classroom can be quite productive. A student not following an established classroom routine would be tantamount to breaking a cultural norm such as moving in front of someone in line at a movie theater. Once embedded in the classroom culture, routines will be assumed and maintained by the students.

✻ ✻ ✻

Routines for Frequent Necessities

The students were working independently on a textbook assignment in Mr. Taylor's class. Mr. Taylor was walking among them providing brief assistance to individuals. Two students rose from their seats, walked to a shelf containing dictionaries at the side of the room, and each took a dictionary from it, as if this were part of an established routine for finding the definitions of unknown words. The students had no need to occupy Mr. Taylor's time, time used for assisting other students. Mr. Taylor did not need to take time to refer them to a dictionary either, as they already knew the routine for acquiring the definitions of unknown words.

A teacher would be wise to examine the most common behaviors students enact daily and consider establishing routines for them. For example, in most classes, students regularly need to sharpen their pencils. However, in many classrooms, especially secondary ones, no routine exists for this task. The noise generated from a pencil sharpener is an auditory distraction to learning and often the beginning of unproductive conversations. The noise generated seems to liberate the students' natural propensity to converse. Establishing a routine such as having the students place a sharpened pencil at the top of their desks prior to the beginning bell, exchanging a sharpened pencil with a student's dull one, or having students use a pen if their pencil needs sharpening during instruction would eliminate the distractions normally associated with pencil sharpening. The following episodes illustrate further the need for establishing a routine for this frequent student behavior.

Mr. Unkershen implemented a counting procedure in response to some mild conversations at the beginning of class and his students became quiet and ready to receive further instruction. However, at that moment, a student rose, walked to the pencil sharpener, and proceeded to sharpen his pencil. The mild conversations resurfaced.

Ms. Villa provided her students with an independent assignment, which involved distinguishing a root from a base. The students were silent and engaged when a student proceeded to the pencil sharpener and sharpened his pencil. This, of course produced a loud distraction. In turn, two students began to converse at a volume that apparently began to worry one student as he responded, "Shhh." Another student proceeded to sharpen his pencil. A different student began to talk and another student exclaimed, "Don't." A student sitting toward the back of the room quietly sounded jokingly, "Ya, ya, ya."

✻ ✻ ✻

Instructional Routines

Mr. Xavier announced to his class, "Would you take out your Cornell notes from yesterday?" He continued, "Alright. Take out another piece of paper." The students followed this directive and began to fold their papers in a distinct manner, in preparation for this note-taking method. No instruction preceded this folding process, as it was apparently part of the routine for taking notes.

After roll call, Mr. Yates announced, "Warm up" to his PE class. Immediately the students sat on their numbers. He then provided brief directives to the students to complete specific movements, "Hands up," "Hands down," "Stand up," "Right over left," "Left over right." Almost all students readily complied. Mr. Yates revealed, "Routines and procedures each day" were key to maintaining an effective learning environment. He added, "Each day you do the same thing. At the end of the period we will return back to the numbers."

Routines suited to a teacher's instructional goals provide the conditioning necessary for a behavior to become a class norm. Once routines are established, behaviors consistent with learning goals become automatic and immune to other distractions. Substitute teachers always want to substitute in a classroom that has solid routines established.

✳ ✳ ✳

Dismissal Routines

Mr. Zane was explaining an assignment to the class when the bell rang, "These are all cities. You get to label the names of the countries. As you write the names, try to say them in Spanish [the dismissal bell sounded]. . . . Gee. Was that the bell? I guess I miscalculated." The students remained seated and placed their belongings in their backpacks. Next, they stood at the side of their desks and waited. Mr. Zane made some final announcements and provided a verbal cue to which the students responded, "Hasta manana." Mr. Zane replied, "Hasta manana," and the students left.

Implementing a dismissal routine promotes engagement through the end of the period. Disengagement prior to the end of class is a common phenomenon but less appealing to students if they know they must engage in the routine prior to being dismissed. Desiring to leave a crowded room is natural and must be considered while maintaining order. Having a routine to guide departure will provide a nice expected cue at the end of class and make dismissal time non-negotiable.

✳ ✳ ✳

Material Distribution/Collection

Mr. Alexander was making some preliminary announcements to his students prior to administering an exam. The students had their tests facing downward, as this was part of the test taking routine. Mr. Alexander announced, "You have plenty of time today and tomorrow to take the test. Take your time. Always work wisely. Show work. Questions?" A student asked, "Number line?" Mr. Alexander replied, "There is a number line. You weren't supposed to turn your paper over yet, were you?" He added, "Any other questions? . . . If you come to a problem you don't know, skip it . . . Good luck." The class remained attentive throughout his introduction. The students then turned over their papers and began working.

Toward the end of the period Mr. Alexander briefly reviewed the procedure for collecting exams, "Okay, to make it easier to pass back tomorrow . . . Scratch paper underneath. If I don't have your names on your papers, it will be too hard to pass back." The students, remaining seated, methodically passed their tests forward with the scratch papers underneath.

In most classrooms, students use a variety of materials, especially paper materials. Paper, for example, is used for exams, essay writing, assignments, taking notes, and organizing.

Routines for arranging these materials save time and provide organization to potentially voluminous material.

* * *

Entering Routines

Mrs. Bently directed her students to prepare a notebook for writing prior to the beginning bell. When the bell sounded she raised both hands and her students raised their notebooks. Mrs. Bently simply asked the students to begin writing and the students complied. Little prompting was necessary to get the students to begin writing, as this was also part of their beginning routine. This routine at the beginning of class focused student attention on learning and contributed to an efficient start.

As described earlier in the no assignment section, having a preparation routine for students upon entering the classroom makes learning a part of the classroom's culture, and conditioning of the students. Routines upon entry focus student attention on instruction prior to the beginning bell.

CATEGORY 5 –

RIGID PRACTICES

N el Noddings' description of her high school math
teacher illustrates the rigid approach (Noddings, 1997):

The math teacher, Mr. Shea, still affects my work.
Although I loved him deeply and the affection was, in
later years, reciprocal, I have to face the fact that many
students hated him, and worse, their hatred was at least
understandable – perhaps even justified. He was rigid in
his methods, overly strict in his classroom management
(which made playing tricks on him a great sport). . . . I
think it is clear that Mr. Shea was not a good teacher for
most kids (p. 173).

Rigid practices include intimidation, expressions of anger, and
consequences without regard to the students' emotional state of
being. Moore's observation of a particular classroom teacher
(Moore, 1967) illustrates this approach's attributes. The teacher
threatens, "From now on you come up with your row or you
won't get what I'm giving out [in reference to a polio shot
permission form]" (p. 135), yells, "'You're not paying
attention,' she shouts at Billy" (p. 137), uses sarcasm, "I've
finished the third row. Where were you when I called on your
row? Have you got two ears on your head?" (p. 135), and

demeans, "Miss Tobins' boys ought to hang their heads in shame, they put on a disgusting performance" (p. 130).

These types of practices have been shown to have devastating effects on children. Moore (1967) indicates that the students of the teacher described above showed "no joy of being taught" (p. 147). He adds that although overly demanding teachers might be getting the material across, "the essential step of learning to learn is not being taken" (p. 146). Cunningham and Sugawara (1989) in their review of disciplinary strategies also found that verbal reprimand, denying privileges, and corporal punishment, have undesirable effects on children over time (Brophy, 1983; Moore & Cooper, 1984; Elliott, Witt, Galvin, & Peterson, 1984). Brophy and Evertson (1981) found that teachers, who highly criticize perceived low level students, publicly compare them unfavorably to others in the class as bad examples, refuse to acknowledge initiations and requests from them, and convey nonverbally feelings of impatience or negative affect generate a high tendency for a negative self fulfilling prophecy effect to occur. Brophy (1983) concludes that students of teachers who use these techniques show a sullen or defiant attitude when teachers attempt to criticize or discipline. He adds that the effort and output of some students is decreased by criticism. Additionally, Traynor (2002) showed that a coercive, task oriented environment obstructs the production of projects at the higher level of Bloom's taxonomy.

Manifesting a more austere disposition is unlikely to gain the compliance consistent with learning. Collette and Chiapette (1989) state that teachers who are unable to control themselves in the long run lose student respect. They add that once students recognize that things are not under control, they are apt to create more problems that incite further misbehavior. Walker, Colvin and Ramsey (1995) further confirm that a student in an agitated state clearly exhibiting maladaptive behavior is likely to continue to escalate the behavior if the teacher continues to argue, use sarcasm, or threaten (p.80).

According to Figure 1, teachers strongly identified with the rigid approach have difficulty avoiding this category of practices.

CHAPTER

22 Unrealistic Expectations

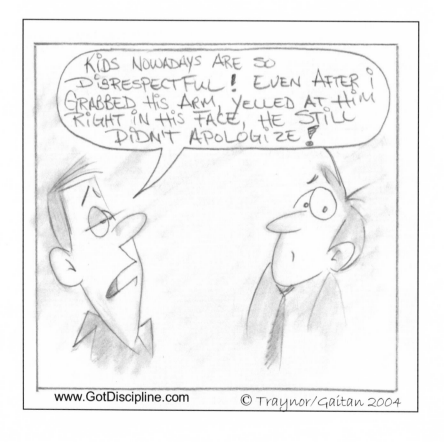

A student entered Mr. Carnegie's class without a pencil or paper. However, one of the classroom rules is to come to class prepared. Mr. Carnegie sent this student to the office with a referral document to the school's administrator of discipline, "Totally unprepared to do any work. No notebook, no pen or pencil, no handbook. Unable to work in class."

Mr. Decker, was seated on the stool at the front of the room. He had recently finished reviewing material on which his students were to be tested. Mr. Decker threatened a student who was talking, "Tommy, do you want zeroes on that?" Another boy began to plea, "He was just asking. . ." Mr. Decker interrupted with an angry, loud tone, "Do I care what he was asking?"

Traynor (2003) showed that when expectations for student behavior do not match a teacher's actual experiences, teachers react to the immediacy of the crowd rather than strategically enact pedagogically sound practices.

This is consistent with a fundamental brain hypothesis, the Triune Brain. According to this hypothesis, the human brain can be divided into three parts, the hypothalamus, the limbic system, and the neocortex. The hypothalamus is designed for protection from bodily harm. When an animal experiences stress, the hypothalamus initiates a sequence of nerve cell firing and chemical release that prepares the animal body for running or fighting. This portion of the brain has been imperative for animal survival where fleeing from or fighting an attacker has been a natural occurrence. When this response is initiated, rational thought from the neocortex is postponed until the animal perceives to be safe and secure.

Expecting students to come to class already with the behaviors consistent with learning is unrealistic. Teachers with this expectation are likely to experience stress more frequently when encountering even minor disruptions. Such teachers will obviously have greater difficulty applying logic when reacting to these encounters, as the fight or flight sequence has already been initiated. A teacher who anticipates maladaptive behavior and realizes the need to teach the behaviors consistent with learning, will experience less stress and be better prepared to enact the appropriate, effective practices described in earlier sections.

CHAPTER

23 Low Empathy

A student fell and hurt his hand. He asked Mr. Easton if he could go to the nurse's office. Rather than sending the student or at least showing concern toward him, Mr. Easton directed him to wait until the end of the period.

A girl approached Mr. Fredrick asking him for assistance. She informed him that she purchased a new ruler and did not know how to read it for her exam. Mr. Fredrick responded, "This is a testing situation, I would expect you to know your materials right now."

Having empathy with students in need promotes interactions that contribute to the maintenance of a classroom climate that promotes fairness and respect. Not having empathy does the opposite. Demonstrating empathy amidst the enormous demands placed on a teacher in the classroom is a skill that is developed and honed throughout one's career. Although demonstrating empathy toward someone who does not reciprocate can be difficult, teachers must realize that few students have experienced situations that require the organization, professional poise, and responsibility of a classroom teacher. Many students do not yet have the necessary background to have such empathy. The more a teacher models empathy and respect, the more likely it is to be learned. Students learn what the teacher models.

CHAPTER

24

Temper

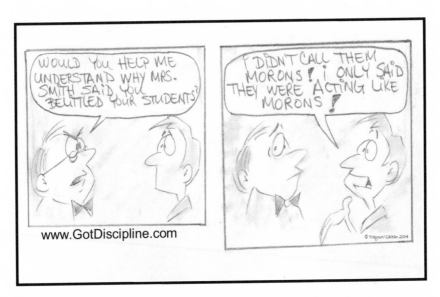

www.GotDiscipline.com

A baseball bat leaned against the wall below the dry erase board. Mr. Gelson disclosed with mild laughter that he uses it for the "intimidation factor." He picked it up to give a demonstration. "I just put it right here and go like that." He hit it on the desk with enough force to make a startling noise. He added, "But I don't do it that much anymore. I just walk around with it once in a while." Toward maintaining order he said, "I may raise my voice to students if they are not paying attention." Mr. Gelson said if the students are being rude to him, returning their rudeness is fair and appropriate. He added that if he did not sometimes yell or return students' rudeness, the class could become unruly. He disclosed that sometimes he will tell them, "Shut your mouth."

Being overly harsh to students has no place in the classroom environment and should in no way be a part of any teacher's repertoire of practices. Students should never have to see a teacher behaving unprofessionally, not under self control, and not in good character. Older students know that harsh, callous behavior demonstrated by a teacher is far worse than even the most detestable student behaviors. A teacher should never say anything to a student that would not be said if the parent were present. Demonstrating severe behavior toward students also greatly increases the likelihood of parent complaints and further hinders the principal's ability to support the teacher in correcting student behavior.

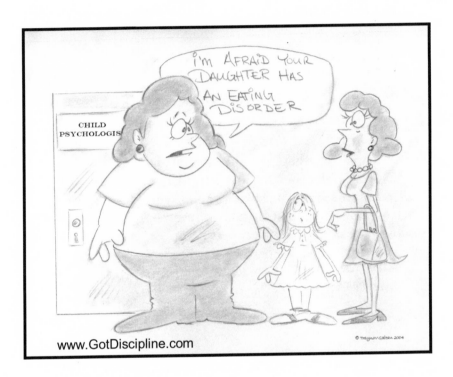

PART III Related Issues

The practices described in Part II occur within the classroom context. However, factors outside of the classroom also must be mentioned as they influence the classroom dynamics considerably. Several of these factors are discussed next.

CHAPTER

25   **Parents**

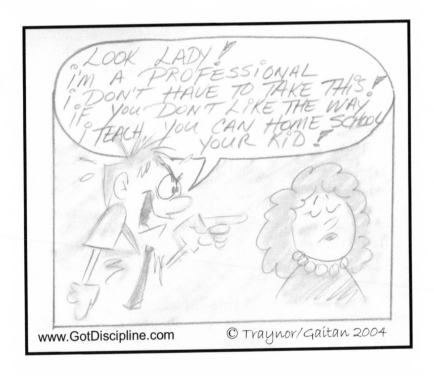

The Telephone as a Proactive Intervention

A student whose parents speak well of the teacher at home is much more likely to demonstrate respect for the teacher inside the classroom. Conversely, students whose parents who do not speak well of the teacher will have difficulty demonstrating respect toward the teacher. When communicating with parents, teachers must always recognize this and strive to maintain parent respect.

One common avenue of communicating with parents is the telephone. When used appropriately, the phone call home can be a teacher's most powerful intervention. Many schools with effective discipline plans require this intervention prior to the disciplinary referral. Saying, "Okay, Johnny, I have warned you, now I will have to call your parents," is often how this intervention begins. Knowing that an evening phone call will be made later, apart from the pressing situation, can provide the teacher with the solace needed to redirect the student's and class' focus on the current lesson in a professional manner.

The first contact with parents should be positive and phone calls home can certainly be used for this purpose. A perceptive and prudent teacher will, on the first day or two of school, identify students who appear likely to test the classroom limits, and make a positive contact with their parents. Fortunately, as described later, the first day or two of school will generally be free of any serious maladaptive behavior, regardless of teacher skill. This makes the first few days a great opportunity to make a positive contact with parents of students who appear likely to misbehave. This practice has two powerful effects: (1) The parent will be pleased to hear positive comments regarding their child and will therefore be more likely to respect this teacher as a professional and communicate this respect for the teacher to the child, and (2) the student in question will understand that the teacher has the fortitude to call the parent at any time. If one takes a closer look, this intervention has even more benefits. A cunning student, when asked to respond to a negative report from a teacher, can claim to be "picked on" or not liked by the teacher. The student can even embellish several examples to support the claim. However, after an early positive parent contact, such a student will realize the opportunity to impart a negative impression of the teacher on the mind of the parent has been greatly diminished. With less opportunity, the student realizes a continuation of maladaptive behavior in the classroom is unlikely to gain support at home. Also, after an initial positive parent contact, the parent is more likely to be supportive of the teacher when the teacher does need to inform the parent of the student's maladaptive behavior in the future. A positive initial contact should sound similar in tone to:

> Hello, I'm Mr. Sacco and I am Johnny's teacher. I just called to introduce myself and I wanted to let you know that I am really looking forward to teaching Johnny this year. Johnny seems like a great young man with a lot of potential and I'm sure you must be really proud of him. I also wanted to let you know that if you have any questions or concerns at any time, please feel free to call me at school. The number is 555-5555. Again, I am really looking forward to teaching Johnny. Have a pleasant evening.

The more specific the teacher can get when making positive comments, the better the impact of this first contact will be.

When a teacher does need to use the phone to inform the parent of maladaptive behavior, the beginning of the conversation should similarly be positive. A teacher could follow the positive comments with the concern about the student. The concern should be related directly to the student's benefit. That is, the teacher should communicate that because the student is behaving poorly, classroom instruction will not be as beneficial or the student might not reach full potential. A teacher should add that if the maladaptive behavior continues, it will interfere with others' learning as well. The phone call should also end with a positive comment about the student.

The maladaptive behavior should be stated precisely. The statement to the parent, "Johnny said to me, 'You sit down,' after I told him to remain in his seat," will gain much more support than the statement, "Johnny has been misbehaving in class." A general or vague statement will leave the parent wanting to know what specifically their child did. This is only right. A teacher should leave the parent on rock solid footing if the parent chooses to implement consequences at home. Not being able to provide specifics reinforces a child's claim of being "picked on" or not liked.

If the phone call is the first contact in which maladaptive behavior is communicated to the parent, the teacher should simply state the steps that will be taken if the behavior does not improve and not make any recommendations. This avoids the perception that the teacher is shifting the responsibility of correcting classroom behavior to the parent. Suggestions of what the parent can do at home might elicit defensive behaviors. As mentioned earlier, the teacher must maintain strong parent support. If this is one of several phone calls, the teacher may inform the parent of the next step, which will likely result in a referral to the administrator of discipline. An intervention phone call home should sound similar in tone to:

> Hello, this is Mr. Sacco. I want to let you know Johnny is a wonderful boy with a lot of potential. He is a pleasure to have in class. The reason I am calling is that I know Johnny could be doing much better. For example, today he refused to stay seated after I told him to stay seated for this assignment. He actually told me to sit down instead. I am afraid that if he continues to disobey our classroom procedures, and defy my authority, his learning will suffer and infringe on the other students' learning. I just want to let you know that I gave him a behavior essay to complete and issued him a detention during recess. The next time Johnny does

this I will have to give him a time out of our classroom and may even need to send him to the office. I don't want to do that. He is such a good boy and has so much potential. Thank you for all your support.

Teachers must not under use this powerful intervention. Often teachers say, "I would call home but it doesn't do any good." This is a myth promulgated by teachers who wish to avoid parent confrontation. When used effectively, the overwhelming majority of parent contacts will be positive and will have a significant impact on changing behavior of most students. Even if this intervention does not work for a particular student and parent, others will ask the student if the teacher followed through with the call. If this student responds affirmatively, even if the response is similar to, "Yeah, Mr. Sacco called. But my parents think he's a jerk anyway," the teacher will gain a reputation for having the fortitude to follow through with consequences and call parents – a powerful reputation to have. Most students will make great efforts to avoid a negative parent report from a teacher.

What if the parents are not home? A message can be left on the answering machine. An organized teacher will log the date with the initials, L.M. (Left Message) next to the student's name on the attendance list or elsewhere. Although, a savvy student can erase the message before the parent hears it, a brief log of the message will serve a teacher well if in the future the parent asks, "Why is this the first time I have heard about this." The teacher can then retrieve the log and say, I left a message on your phone on [date], I am sorry you did not receive it." The parent should realize that their child has been insubordinate at home and be more likely to support a teacher's accusations that Johnny indeed has the propensity to engage in maladaptive behavior. Further, a child who has erased a message is more likely to want to avoid another parent contact in which the teacher will certainly recall the prior phone message.

What about parents who do not have a phone? A simple way to communicate is to write a note to give to the student to take home. Similar to leaving a message, a teacher can log the date the note was given to the student with the initials, S.N. (Sent Note) next to the student's name. A teacher who has a computer with a printer in the classroom can efficiently accomplish this task while retaining a copy. Of course the same information that would be included in the phone call or answering machine message will not be on a note; a simple statement of facts will be effective. A brief written message should be similar in form to, "Today, Johnny refused to sit down in his seat and told me, 'You sit down.' I have given him a detention and a behavior essay. Please call if you have any questions, 555-5555." Notes can also be mailed. Although school procedures may vary, the school secretaries and office staff are accustomed to mailing letters and mailing a letter home for a teacher should be a simple matter of routine.

What about parents who do not speak English? America is becoming more linguistically diverse with people who do not have ready access to the English language. If a school has a designated bilingual liaison for this purpose, a phone call home can be even more powerful. A parent who does not speak English generally feels alienated from the people who do. If they hear someone speaking their language, they immediately feel validated – someone has gone to the trouble to communicate with them; they are important. A tactful bilingual staff member can communicate with the parents who do not speak English in the manner described above. The same bilingual staff member can also leave answering machine messages and write notes to parents in the manner described above.

As more phones are being installed inside classrooms, one common practice has been to direct students who exhibit maladaptive behavior to call home and explain the incident before the class. This practice has the pitfalls associated with both the lenient and the rigid category of practices. Giving up too much control over the communication by having the student call the parent allows the student to lighten the magnitude of the maladaptive behavior and has the negative effects consistent with the lenient disposition (see lenient disposition described above). Also, directing students to speak in front of peers about their own maladaptive behavior is potentially humiliating and has the negative effects consistent with the rigid disposition (see rigid disposition section above). Parents might also wonder why the teacher is not calling them directly and lose respect for the teacher. Parent respect, as described above, is a powerful asset toward maintaining student respect.

❋ ❋ ❋

Returning Calls

If a teacher should receive a telephone message from a parent, being prompt in returning the call is vital to maintaining a professional image. Returning the call within 24-hours is the professional standard. Not returning the call elicits complaints to administration. If a teacher wishes to solve the problem without administrative intervention or documentation (a phone message regarding a complaint), a prompt return will certainly be advantageous.

Also, knowing the parent's concern prior to returning the call will be helpful toward gathering information for reference. If the teacher believes the parent wishes to know more about how a low grade was given, a grade book with all assignments listed would be helpful. If the teacher suspects a child misinterpreted a particular communication, knowing what to say to the parent prior to the phone call will contribute to a productive interaction. Saying, "I am sorry, I did not mean to communicate that [whatever the child understood]. What I meant was [whatever was intended to be communicated]," would serve a teacher well in rectifying a concern.

Hearing defensive comments from a teacher is often perceived from a parent's perspective as "The teacher feels justified in everything said and done and does not value what I have to say." Unfortunately many teachers perceive apologizing or acknowledging a legitimate viewpoint of a parent as damaging to their pride. Teachers are professionals and should always view themselves as professionals. Arguing with a parent, regardless of how correct a teacher is, seldom enhances the parent's perception of the teacher, or helps the situation. Teachers should not let false pride hinder professional, appropriate communication, and should apologize when an apology is warrented. Listening to the parent's concern and responding with what will happen in the future, even if it is following the same procedure, routine, etc., already in place, will serve to assure the parent that the teacher understands the problem and is responsive. The teacher does not need to admit, deny or respond to allegations.

Providing a follow-up call after a problem has been solved is an outstanding way to gain parent support. First, parents do not expect the caliber of service characteristic of a high quality business. Second, calling back after a teacher has rectified a situation will usually be met with sincere gratitude. Third, knowing that a follow up call will be made provides the teacher with a self-induced incentive to solve the problem.

❋ ❋ ❋

Parent Conferences

Conferences provide another medium for parent and teacher interaction. Frequently parent conferences are built into the school's yearly calendar. Parent conferences are opportunities to build positive parent support, not to surface concerns about student behavior that should have been addressed prior to the conference. Staying objective and focused on achievement data and emphasizing the student's strengths will set a professional tone for the conference. If unpleasant information needs to be communicated, the teacher must do this diplomatically, for example, ". . . and if Johnny only worked a little harder on his spelling words, his spelling scores would increase tremendously. Also, if he knew his math facts, he would not be struggling so much with these math assignments." If the parents ask what Johnny could be doing to improve, disclosing the improper behavior at that moment would be appropriate. Again, the teacher should relate the concern to the student's benefit, for example, "If Johnny was more compliant, he would be making better progress." This is much better than simply saying, "Johnny consistently defies my authority." Although predicting the direction of all possible dialogues is impossible, keeping a professional attitude and a positive tone while communicating necessary information will serve a teacher well in gaining parent support. The author has seen this first hand on many occasions.

❋ ❋ ❋

Addressing Concerns

In the business community, organizations compete for, need, and appreciate customer business. Organization and customer interactions must leave a positive image the mind of the customer in order for the organization to thrive. Employees that communicate directly with the organization's customers have a powerful effect on shaping the organization's image.

Similar to organizations in the private sector, teachers would do well for their own image as well as the school's by addressing all concerns in a reasonable, professional manner. Parent concerns usually arise from a child's description of an incident, a particular interaction, a calculation of an overall grade, a score on a particular project, etc. Parents usually become aware of the problem first by hearing the context of the situation described from their child's perspective. Some students even embellish the facts to make their point. If the teacher was wrong, partially wrong, or could reasonably

ameliorate a parent's concern, the teacher should certainly do
so. More often than not, the result will be an amicable solution
to the problem. If the teacher gets defensive, remains inflexible,
or unwilling to consider a parent's perspective, a negative image
can be imprinted on the mind of the parent. On the other hand,
if a concern is solved professionally, amicably, and within
reasonable limits, a particularly positive image is likely to be
imprinted. A teacher should view the concern from the parent's
perspective, empathize, and offer a reasonable solution.
Keeping the end goal in mind – student learning for the
student's benefit – will provide focus to problem solving
discussions.

Unfortunately, some parents push the limits of what is
acceptable and threaten to complain to the principal, pull their
child out of class, or even go to superintendent or the local
school board meeting to voice their concern. If the teacher has
offered a reasonable solution (and hopefully the teacher is
willing to be part of a reasonable solution), a confident
statement such as the following can deflect such a threat:

> That's fine, that's your choice. You may go to the
> principal, district office, or board to complain. What
> they will do is make certain that I am responding to your
> concern in a reasonable manner. Is there anything in
> what I am proposing that you find unreasonable and
> would like changed? I am committed to doing what is
> reasonable.

The teacher should be positive. Focusing on what can be done
rather than what cannot be done keeps the parent's attention on
reasonable solutions. Stating what cannot be done, even if the
parent has brought it up, gives many parents a feeling that a
more satisfactory solution is available but will not be offered.

Although many complaints can be deflected in the
manner described above, compromising high and reasonable
standards must not be an option to appease parent concerns. A
teacher, who is genuinely imparting knowledge and mastery of

higher level learning objectives, simply will not please everyone. However, a teacher, who has worked toward a reasonable solution, in a professional and positive manner, should feel confident regardless of what an unsatisfied parent threatens. Brief documentation of the steps taken toward ameliorating the concern should provide the teacher with added security – proof that a reasonable solution involving the parent was developed.

CHAPTER

26   **ADHD**

> One of the hardest things is going out to casual get-togethers where people are not tolerant or understanding or knowledgeable about it [ADHD]. Many times I have left events and cried on the way home because people have commented about how "bad" Alan was. They expect children to sit and be quiet.
>
> Parent

The practices in this book most certainly apply to the supervision of children with Attention Deficit Hyperactivity Disorder (ADHD). The major difference is that with an ADHD student, more frequent interventions and a more moderate disposition are needed. Not all students will be able to sit still and "engage" in the prescribed daily content standards, regardless of how strongly managed.

The following interventions (except the last two – Medication and Realistic Expectations) were adapted with permission from the U.S. Department of Education – Office of Special Education Programs publication (2004).

✻ ✻ ✻

Verbal Reinforcement

Providing specific and positive praise for desired behavior is effective for all students and is especially effective for ADHD students. The comments should focus on what the student did right and should include exactly what part(s) of the student's behavior was desirable. Rather than praising a student for not disturbing the class, for example, a teacher should provide praise for quietly completing a math lesson on time. Providing this praise immediately increases the likelihood that the student will repeat it. Sincere praise additionally increases the effectiveness of the praise. Varying the praise maintains a genuine appearance.

The most effective teachers focus their behavioral intervention strategies on praise rather than on punishment. Negative consequences may temporarily change behavior, but they rarely change attitudes and may actually increase the frequency and intensity of inappropriate behavior by rewarding misbehaving students with attention. Moreover, punishment teaches children what not to do and does not reinforce skills. Positive reinforcement produces the changes in attitudes that will shape a student's behavior over the long term.

✳ ✳ ✳

Selectively Ignoring Inappropriate Behavior

As discussed in the Indirect Interventions portion of this book, selectively ignoring inappropriate behavior can often allow the behavior to extinguish itself. This technique is particularly useful when the behavior is unintentional or unlikely to recur or is intended solely to gain the attention of teachers or classmates.

✳ ✳ ✳

Teaching Self Management

Children with ADHD should be explicitly taught appropriate social skills. This can be done by role-playing or modeling different solutions to common social problems. Providing structured practice opportunities will allow the child to develop skill in applying the specific behavior in a variety of settings, inside and outside of class.

Explicitly teaching students specific formats for resolving conflicts will provide the student with a functional as opposed to maladaptive device for solving minor conflicts. One format the author has seen used effectively called generically here, the "Conflict Solving Process," consists of three steps. The first is to directly communicate to the other person exactly what is desired – for example, "Would you please let me take a turn?" The second step is used if the first step did not work. It consists of simply restating the request and naming the appropriate adult that will be involved next, for example, "Would you please let me take a turn or I am telling Mrs. McGill? The final step is taken if the second step did not work. It is simply following through with the second step – telling the appropriate adult. The adult in turn can ask the child if the "Conflict Solving Process" was used. If not, guiding the child through each step can be especially instructional.

✳ ✳ ✳

Environmental Considerations

As mentioned with the indirect interventions, the physical environment can prepared ahead of time to facilitate productive order. Removing nuisance items such as rubber bands and toys is generally most effective after the student has been given the choice of putting the item(s) away immediately and then fails to do so.

Seating the child close to the teacher or to a positive peer role model can promote proper behavior. Seating the child near the teacher provides opportunities to monitor and reinforce the child's on-task behavior. Seating the child near a student role model provides an opportunity to work cooperatively and to learn from peers in the class.

Setting a timer to indicate to children how much time remains in the lesson provides an impending feeling of relief, especially with monotonous tasks. Placing the timer at the front of the classroom allows the children to check how much time remains. Interim prompts can be used as well. For instance, children can monitor their own progress during a 30-minute lesson if the timer is set for 10 minutes three times.

Allowing an ADHD child to manifest the "condition" will make the child's environment more "natural." For example, permitting the child to leave class for a moment on an errand, such as returning a book to the library, will provide the child with relief from the restrictive, artificial classroom environment that is full of many barriers.

✳ ✳ ✳

Medication

For parents, the use of medication for their child is controversial. Many parents correctly argue that taking medication for ADHD is not natural. However, what is expected of kids inside a classroom is not natural. Societal norms exceed human evolutionary capacity. As stated in the introduction, behaving orderly in large groups under the direction of an unfamiliar adult in tight quarters is not natural. However, this is a school norm. A student who is diagnosed with ADHD is at a great disadvantage in the classroom's artificial setting. Forcing an ADHD parent to decide whether or not to medicate their child for school is unfortunate. All medications have side effects and parents should be encouraged to consult a physician on the issue. Although the cause of ADHD remains unknown, research suggests a neurobiological basis. In many instances, medication, under a doctor's prescription, leads to more productive ADHD students.

Great deference should be given to a parent's choice in this matter. At a parent conference, one teacher told a parent to consider increasing the dose of medication for their child as a remedy for making the child's behavior more endurable in class.

The parent later disclosed in frustration, "I think the teacher needs to take medication to increase his tolerance of children."

❊ ❊ ❊

Realistic Expectations

Still, even with medication, the teacher should expect the ADHD student to require much more attention than the average student. As stated earlier, realistic expectations are associated with enacting strategies the teacher knows are pedagogically sound (Traynor, 2003). Unrealistic expectations are associated with stress, invoke the fight or flight reflex, and prevent the teacher from acting rationally. The U. S. Office of Special Education states that ADHD students "frequently fail to finish their schoolwork, or they work carelessly" (2004). One of their prescriptions is to "help students focus. Remind students to keep working and to focus on their assigned task." (p.7). Simply expecting an ADHD student to stay seated, stay on task, and follow structured classroom procedures and routines without frequent prompting is unrealistic. Although an ADHD student should not consume all of the teacher's time, additional prompting, reminding, and intervening should be expected.

Finally, ADHD does not mean low capability. ADHD students frequently outperform classmates. They also have the capacity to be just as respectful. However, too often, they are not viewed as students who are bright and respectful, but as students who are "having trouble" that must be "disciplined." Knowing that the wiggles, tendencies to be off-task, and expressions of frustration when doing mundane work are not fully controllable, will prepare the teacher for more realistic expectations.

In fact, ADHD can be argued to have a positive aspect. Anne Underwood (2005) describes two books (*Delivered from Distraction* by Dr. Edward Hallowell and Dr. John Ratey, and *The Gift of ADHD* by Dr. Lara Hones-Webb, a psychologist from Santa Clara University) that advance the "notion that distractibility, poor impulse control, and emotional sensitivity have flip sides that are actually strengths – namely creativity, energy, and intuition" (p. 48). Underwood cites Hones-Webb, who describes the ADHD mind as being able to excel at combining ideas in new ways, "While the A students are learning the details of photosynthesis, the ADHD kids are staring out the window and wondering if it still works on a cloudy day" (p. 48).

CHAPTER

27   **Antisocial Behavior**

E very day teachers have contact with students who are on the verge of exhibiting tantrum-like behavior. Although most students come to school with a predisposition to behave in a socially appropriate manner (not yell, threaten, or tantrum), any student has the potential to break social bounds and escalate minor maladaptive behavior into more severe behavior. Walker, Colvin, and Ramsey (1995) found that children with antisocial behavior have a tendency to "act out" according to a seven sequence chain of behavior phases with the fifth phase being the most severe. If not careful, a teacher can inadvertently trigger the onset of this chain and continue to escalate the child's behavior to a higher phase. The phases of higher intensity are much more difficult to manage as they include tantrums, yelling, throwing, and even physical assault. When an incident is in its primary phases, the child's behavior is still manageable. Educators must be aware that certain students, under certain conditions, enter the classroom already in what is called a "triggered" state, phase 2, in which a seemingly calm student can be easily agitated. Any form of a direct confrontation, explicit directive, or irritating stimuli can escalate latent behavior into a higher phase of the cycle (p. 80-81).

Diffusing the anger in a student who is escalating the maladaptive behavior should be a top priority. A skillful teacher will be able to identify such a student and momentarily suspend any type of learning demands. Although usually the student will not pose a physical threat to anyone inside the classroom, the goal of the teacher is to keep this student as least disruptive as possible and avoid escalation. The time for counseling should be later, when the student is able to think and act rationally.

After recognizing that a student is in the "triggered" state or higher phase of the acting out behavior cycle, the teacher may use one of a variety of techniques such as providing appropriate, peaceful space, a preferred activity, or relaxation activities. Nurturing practices described above, strategic avoidance, and remaining calm and professional will also serve a teacher well to diffuse the behavior. Physical restraint of the child should only be used if physical injury to anyone in the environment is imminent. If it is used, the teacher should report this to the administration as soon as possible with follow up documentation. Teachers should view challenges like these as opportunities to model professionalism and caring for the rest of the class.

Although any student has the potential to exhibit tantrum like behaviors, generally speaking, if any one student has three or more episodes in one month, a pattern is established, and formal action must be taken. This includes a documented meeting to develop interventions. The meeting should include the teacher and other staff who service the student, such as a counselor, an administrator, and a parent. Alternative, replacement behavior patterns that are adaptive and functional can be taught by direct teaching, behavior management methods, positive and negative consequences, and providing access to counseling (Walker, Colvin, and Ramsey, 1995; pp 130-136).

CHAPTER

28   The First Day

As discussed earlier, the first few moments of class set the learning tone for the period or day. Similarly, the first day of school sets the learning tone for the year. If the first day is well organized, structured learning is provided, and behaviors consistent with learning are maintained, these behaviors are more likely to become established. The teacher then need only focus on maintenance for the remainder of the year. Too often teachers try to "break the ice," do not spend enough time preparing the learning for the day, and unwittingly think that since the kids are behaving well the first few days, that discipline will not be an issue for them that year.

Providing a clear, structured lesson in which all students will engage is appropriate. At the secondary level in particular, providing a short diagnostic test that assesses student knowledge and skill from the moment they enter sets a nice learning tone those precious first few moments of the year. The test, of course, would be without penalty and contain several questions of different complexity ranging from simple to difficult. The goal here is to keep students focused on learning while the teacher directs them to their seats as they enter, attends to student questions, and solves any other problems that arise.

Regardless of what exercise the teacher chooses, the precious first minutes at the beginning of the year must not be tainted with distractions that spoil the students' conditioning. A prudent teacher heeds the adage, "You never get a second chance to make a first impression." Many successful educators are aware of these precious moments. Harry and Rosemary Wong (1998) even wrote a 338 page book on the subject, *The First Days of School*.

CHAPTER

29 The Disciplinary Referral

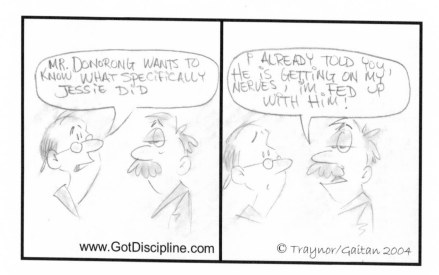

A disciplinary referral to the office should be used only when the teacher has exhausted all interventions. It should not be part of a teacher's regular practice. As a rule, referrals should not be written if the teacher knows the student's behavior could be corrected with a little more effort. If a teacher regularly writes referrals to the office, the symbolic impact of "the office" rapidly diminishes, and the teacher will lose credibility not only with the administrative staff, but with students and parents as well. The first parent contact regarding a student's behavior must not come from the administration. However, if a teacher's nurturing, indirect, and direct practices fail to improve maladaptive behavior, and parent contacts and other interventions have also failed, a referral to the administrator of discipline is necessary. A student should not be allowed to destroy the learning environment for the rest of the students.

Referrals should include all, or most significant interventions applied such as time out within the classroom, time out during recess or lunch, behavior or reflection essay, phone calls home, after school detentions, etc. These might be items that can be checked off on the disciplinary referral itself. Usually referral forms contain a space for a brief narrative. Only the facts should be disclosed – that is, what the student did, not what the teacher thinks the child was intending to do, or how the teacher thinks the child was feeling. A teacher may include the tone in which a child's statement was made. However, this can even be misinterpreted. The more inarguable a teacher can make the statements on the referral, the better. The closer a teacher can stay factual, the better. Any opinion listed is likely to be used as evidence that the teacher is picking on the student, even if the opinion is totally valid and the student has clearly demonstrated a pattern of unacceptable behavior. If opinions do not have to be added to the referral, they should not. Facts listed on a referral document speak for themselves. Opinions make the teacher the adversary. For example, "Johnny was argumentative, disrespectful, and was disturbing the rest of the class," is much more judgmental and less effective than, "After being prompted to remain seated, Johnny said to me, 'You sit down,' and continued to speak out without raising his hand despite warnings."

As stated above in the parent section, once a teacher begins to sense maladaptive behavior becoming established in a student, the teacher should contact the parent. Also as stated above, the first contact with a student's parent should be positive. A parent of a behaviorally challenged child has likely received many more negative contacts from the school system than positive through the years and is therefore apt to be defensive if confronted with disagreeable information.

Further, a teacher should know that children, who reach the point where maladaptive behavior appears intractable, usually have stories of their own background that would bring many to tears. Any school counselor with experience in inner city school districts knows this to be true. Knowing this should inspire patience and a few more interventions before giving up.

PART IV Justification for Managing Behavior

A fundamental premise of this book is that actively maintaining behaviors consistent with learning is necessary for learning to occur in today's classrooms. Some discount this premise arguing that students must first understand why they need to be managed and accept the reasoning in order to grow intellectually and ethically. They claim if students genuinely understand why appropriate behavior is necessary, they would collectively demonstrate behaviors consistent with learning.

For example, Sarason (1990) argues that students should have a role in defining power relationships in the classroom and in implementing power. This, he asserts will "instill in students an understanding of a commitment to the classroom constitution, and an awareness that their opinions will be respected, even if not accepted" (p. 86). Alfie Kohn (1996) writes, "The more we 'manage' students' behavior and try to make them do what we say, the more difficult it is for them to become morally sophisticated people who think for themselves and care about others" (p. 62).

Their conviction that maturing students, even in confined space, have a natural inclination to form and abide by a classroom constitution, respect one another, and demonstrate the behaviors consistent with learning fits nicely with a homogeneous Western European middle class learning community. However, it does not fit current reality in America where cultural diversity is a significant characteristic. Diversity brings different values, beliefs, and assumptions of how one should behave in a classroom. Diaz-Rico and Weed (2002), in their explanation of how students of different cultures must adjust, put forth, "It may take time – and explicit coaching – for students to learn the set of behaviors appropriate for a U.S. school context" (p. 62). Not being aware of or understanding this diversity and assuming today's students automatically come to school with Western European middle class behaviors are counterproductive in managing today's classroom.

Not only is cultural diversity a reality, accountability toward student mastery of content standards is part of America's current ideology. Examples of this include No Child Left Behind with Adequate Yearly Progress and Annual Measurable Objectives, high school exit exams, student retention laws, and accompanying federal and state penalties including state takeover of schools if standardized test scores do not soar. Ignoring today's accountability legislation is not useful toward leading students toward accomplishing school goals.

Demonstrating intrinsic motivation toward mastering these content standards is certainly not a universal student trait inside classrooms. As put forth above, students in groups have a natural propensity toward disorder (see not occupying students' time, not monitoring, and monitoring sections). They enter confined quarters, sit in small desks, and access materials and a variety of information from their textbooks, teachers, computers, handouts, etc. They will not spontaneously engage in an inquiry-based discussion on how they should organize themselves. They need clear direction with strong authority. Those who espouse otherwise might become more enlightened if they supervised school lunch-time activities, bus loading, a school dance, or substitute-teach.

Gutek (1997) affirms, "When educators are unable to recognize the philosophical and ideological perspectives from which proposals emanate, they are unable either to criticize or to implement these proposals from a professional perspective" (p. 9). The proposals or practices in this book emanate from (1) society's current rigorous student performance expectations, (2) the need for students with diverse backgrounds to adjust to behaviors consistent with learning in U.S. classrooms, and (3) the tendency for large groups of youngsters toward disorder in undersized rooms. The effective and ineffective practices described in this book were taken directly from U.S. classrooms where accountability, diversity, and confined quarters indeed exist. Only if these variables change, would less strategic practices be more appropriate.

Additionally, strong management does not mean coercive practices. The practices described as effective in this book are all humane. Coercive practices should not be a form of power at a teacher's disposal. Teachers are professionals, have a responsibility to manifest their professionalism in their interactions with children, and have a responsibility to exercise authority in a just manner, not only to preserve student dignity, but to model appropriate use of authority as well.

Modeling appropriate behavior and exercising appropriate authority are powerful means of instilling the concepts of the United States' Constitution. Creating a mutually constructed classroom constitution, not intervening to maintain behavior consistent with learning, and simply expecting a large group of students to behave productively toward the creation of a meaningful project, might contribute to new teacher failure. One teacher described in disappointment, an experience when working with some student-teachers:

> I remember a couple of them went to student-teacher classes and they laid out the display and they thought that that is all they had to do was lay out the display and

that the kids would just start naturally asking questions
or be totally consumed by the same topic of interest.

Teachers should not squander the first few moments at the
beginning of the school year developing a mutually agreed upon
classroom constitution. These precious moments should be used
for shaping the behaviors consistent with learning.

Students cannot be deceived into thinking that if they
wanted anarchy, the teacher would allow it. They also have the
capacity to understand the basis of classroom rules if directly
taught. The experience of creating a shared classroom
constitution with fair, consistent, and logical rules could be part
of an excellent social studies unit later in the school year.
However, on the first day of school, instilling expectations and
standards for student behavior is imperative. Behavior in
today's classroom, in today's America, with today's standards,
clearly needs to be managed using appropriate research-based
practices.

APPENDIX

Standard Two – California Standards for the Teaching Profession.

		Levels of Professional Accomplishment			
		Practice Not Consistent with Standard Expectations	Developing Beginning Practice	Maturing Beginning Practice	Experienced Practice that Exemplifies the Standard
Element	2.1 Creating a physical environment that engages all students	The physical environment does not support student learning. There are one or more safety hazards, and materials are difficult to access when needed.	The physical environment is arranged for safety and accessibility, and it facilitates individual student engagement in learning.	The arrangement of the physical environment ensures safety and accessibility. Most students work well individually or together as they participate in learning activities.	The arrangement of the physical environment ensures safety and accessibility, and facilitates constructive interaction and purposeful engagement for all students in learning activities.
	2.2 Establishing a climate that promotes fairness and respect	The classroom climate is characterized by unfairness or disrespect, either between the teacher and students or among students. Students are unwilling to take risks. Teacher response to inappropriate behaviors is unfair or inequitable.	A climate of fairness, caring and respect is established by the teacher for most students, but few students take risks and the teacher does little to encourage them. For the most part, the pattern of teacher response to inappropriate behavior is fair and equitable.	A climate of fairness, caring, and respect is maintained by the teacher, and students are encouraged to take risks and be creative. The pattern of teacher response to inappropriate behavior is fair and equitable.	Students ensure that a climate of equity, caring and respect is maintained in the classroom, and students take risks and are creative. The pattern of teacher response to inappropriate behavior is fair and equitable.
	2.3 Promoting social development and group responsibility	Students' social development, self-esteem, and diversity are not supported, and students have no sense of responsibility for each other.	Students respect each other's differences most of the time and work together moderately well. The teacher provides limited opportunities for students to assume responsibility.	Students respect each other's differences and work independently and collaboratively, taking responsibility for themselves and their peers.	Students work independently and collaboratively and maintain a classroom community in which they respect each other's differences, assume leadership and are responsible for themselves and their peers.
	2.4 Establishing and maintaining standards for student behavior	No standards for behavior appear to have been established, or students are confused about what the standards are.	Standards for behavior have been established by the teacher, and the teacher's response to student behavior is generally appropriate.	Standards for behavior are established, are clear to all students and are maintained by the teachers. The teacher's response to student behavior is appropriate.	Students and teacher develop standards for behavior together and students are responsible for helping each other maintain standards.
	2.5 Planning and implementing classroom procedures and routines that support student learning	Classroom procedures and routines have not been established or are not being enforced.	Procedures and routines have been established and work moderately well with little loss of instructional time.	Procedures and routines work smoothly, with no loss of instructional time.	Students and teacher ensure that the classroom procedures and routines operate seamlessly and efficiently.
	2.6 Using instructional time effectively	Learning activities are often rushed or too long, and transitions are rough or confusing, resulting in a loss of instructional time.	Instructional time is paced so that most students complete learning activities. Transitions used to move students into new activities are generally effective.	Pacing of the lesson is appropriate to the activities and enables all students to engage successfully with the content. Transitions are smooth.	Pacing of the lesson is adjusted as needed to ensure the engagement of all students in learning activities. Transitions are seamless.

BIBLIOGRAPHY

Albert, L. (1996). <u>Cooperative discipline</u>. Circle Pines, Minn: American Guidance Service.

Brint, S. G. (1998). <u>Schools and society</u>. Thousand Oaks: Pine Forge Press.

Brooks, D. M. (1985). "The first day of school." <u>Educational Leadership</u>. May 1985, 76-78.

Brophy, J. (1983). "Research on the self-fulfilling prophecy and teacher expectations." <u>Journal of Educational Psychology,</u> 75, 631-661.

Brophy, J., & Evertson, C. (1981). <u>Student characteristics and teaching</u>. New York: Longman.

Canter, L., & Canter, M. (1992). <u>Assertive discipline: Positive behaviors management for today's classroom</u>. 2d e. Santa Monica, Calif.: Canter & Associates. Charles, C. M. (1999). <u>Building Classroom Discipline.</u> New York: Addison Wesley Longman Company.

Coleman, J. S. , Hoffer, T., & Kilgore, S. (1982). <u>High School Achievement: Public, Catholic and Private Schools Compared</u>. New York: Basic Books

Collette, A. T., & Chiappetta, E. L. (1989). <u>Science instruction in the middle and secondary schools.</u> (2nd Ed.). Columbus: Merril.

Coloroso, B. (1994). <u>Kids are worth it! Giving your child the gift of inner discipline.</u> New York: William Morrow.

Cunningham, B., & Sugawara, A. (1989). "Factors contributing to preservice teachers' management of children's problem behaviors." <u>Psychology in the Schools, 26,</u> 370-379.

Cusick, P. A. (1983). <u>The egalitarian ideal and the American high school: studies of three schools</u>. New York: Longman.

Cusick, P. A. (1992). <u>The educational system: Its nature and logic.</u> New York: McGraw-Hill.

DeMarrais, K. B., LeCompte, M. D. (1999). The way schools work: A sociological analysis of education. Addison Wesley Longman, Inc.

Diaz-Rico, L.T., Weed, K. Z. (2002). The crosscultural, language, and academic development handbook. Boston, MA: Allyn and Bacon

Dreikers, R., Grunwald, B., Pepper, E. (1982). Maintaining sanity in the classroom. New York: Harper and Row.

Elliott, S., Witt, J., Galvin, G., & Peterson, R. (1984). "Acceptability of positive and reductive behavioral interventions: Factors that influence teachers' decision." Journal of School Psychology, 22, 353-360.

Engelmann, S., & Colvin, G. (1983). Generalized compliance training. Austin, TX: PRO-ED.

Gaddy, J. R., & Kelly, L. E. (1984). "Down safe corridors: eliminating school disruption." NASSP Bulletin, 68, 13-17.

Gettinger, M. (1988). "Methods of pro-active classroom management." School Psychology Review, 17, 227-242.

Grant, G. P. (1988). The world we created at Hamilton High. Cambridge: Harvard University Press.

Gutek, G. L. (1997). Philosophical and ideological perspectives on education: Second Edition. Allyn and Bacon.

Jones, F. (2000). Tools for teaching. Santa Cruz, CA. Frederic H. Jones & Associates, Inc.

Kohn, A. (1996). Beyond discipline: From compliance to community. Alexandria, Va.: Association for Supervision and Curriculum Development

Moore, G. A., Jr. (1967). Realities of the urban classroom. Garden City, NY: Anchor Books.

Moore, W., & Cooper, H. (1984). "Correlations between teacher and student background and teacher perceptions of descriptive problems and disciplinary techniques." Psychology in the Schools, 21, 386-392.

Newman, F. M., Rutter, R. A., Smith, M. S. (1989). "Organizational Factors that affect teachers' sense of efficacy, community and expectations." Sociology of Education 62, 221-38.

Noddings, N. (1997). Accident, awareness, and actualization. Learning from our lives: Women, research, and autobiography in education, Danvers, MA: Teachers College, Columbia University.

Sarason, S. B. (1990). The predictable failure of educational reform. Jossey Bass.

Steinberg, L., Dornbush, S. M., & Brown, B. B. (1992). "Ethnic differences in adolescent achievement: An ecological perspective." American Psychologist, 47, (6), 723-729.

Traynor, Patrick L. (2002). "A scientific evaluation of five different strategies teachers use to maintain order." Education, 122, 493-509.

Traynor, Patrick L. (2003). "Factors contributing to teacher choice of classroom order strategies." Education, 123, 586-599.

Traynor, Patrick L. (2004). A study comparing three classroom management approaches. Dissertation on file at the University of California, Riverside.

Underwood, Anne (2005). "The gift of ADHD?" Newsweek March 14, 2005.

U.S. Department of Education, Office of Special Education (2004) Teaching Children with Attention Deficit Hyperactivity Disorder: Instructional Strategies and Practices, Washington, D.C., 2004. www.ed.gov/teachers/needs/speced/adhd/adhd-resource-pt2.pdf.

Walker, H. M., Colvin, G., & Ramsey, E. (1995). Antisocial behavior in school: strategies and best practices. Brooks/Cole Publishing Company.

Wong, H. K., Wong, R. T. (1998). How to be an effective teacher: The first days of school. Harry K. Wong Publications, Inc.

Young, K. R. (1993). "The role of social skills training in the prevention and treatment of behavioral disorders." In B. Smith (Ed.), Focus 1993 – Teaching students with learning and behavioral problems (pp. 341-367). Victoria, British Columbia: Smith.

INDEX

ABOUT THE AUTHOR

Patrick Traynor earned his Ph.D. degree in Educational Administration at the University of California, Riverside. His dissertation was on classroom management. His Bachelor of Science degree was earned at the University of California, Davis and included a double major in Nutrition Science and Entomology. In his over 15 years of experience in the field of education, Dr. Traynor has been a middle school principal, elementary school principal, middle school assistant principal, elementary vice principal, high school science teacher, elementary school teacher, and cub scout den leader and cub master. He is currently Director of Language Support Services in Colton Joint Unified School District in San Bernardino County, California. Dr. Traynor has also been a Lecturer at the University of California, Riverside in the Graduate School of Education. He has been published in the areas of classroom management and instructional technology in educational journals including Education, Journal of Instructional Psychology, Learning and Leading with Technology, and Education California (EdCal). His article, "A Scientific Evaluation of Five Classroom Order Strategies" won the Special Merit Award from the journal, Education, in 2002.

He is married to consulting author Dr. Elizabeth Traynor, a Diplomat of the American Board of Psychiatry and Neurology. She has a private practice in Orange County, California. Dr. Elizabeth Traynor has given talks to the medical community on Adult Attention Deficit Disorder, strokes, and futile care, has served on Saddleback Memorial Hospital's ethics committee, and has been published in the American Academy of Neurology. The Drs. Traynor have two children in the public school system.

If you would like more information on Dr. Patrick Traynor, please visit his website, www.patricktraynor.com or contact him, patricktraynor@patricktraynor.com.